T0195111

## Acute Management of
# Hand
# Injuries

# Acute Management of
# Hand
# Injuries

Andrew J. Weiland, MD
Hospital for Special Surgery
New York, NY

Rachel S. Rohde, MD
William Beaumont Hospital
Royal Oak, MI

*Delivering the best in health care information and education worldwide*
6900 Grove Road · Thorofare, NJ 08086

www.slackbooks.com

ISBN: 978-1-55642-853-1

Copyright © 2009 by SLACK Incorporated

Published by:      SLACK Incorporated
                   6900 Grove Road
                   Thorofare, NJ 08086 USA
                   Telephone: 856-848-1000
                   Fax: 856-848-6091
                   www.slackbooks.com

Contact SLACK Incorporated for more information about other books in this field or about the availability of our books from distributors outside the United States.
Library of Congress Cataloging-in-Publication Data

Weiland, Andrew J.
   Acute management of hand injuries / Andrew J. Weiland, Rachel S. Rohde.
      p. ; cm.
   Includes bibliographical references and index.
   ISBN-13: 978-1-55642-853-1 (alk. paper)
   ISBN-10: 1-55642-853-7 (alk. paper)
   1. Hand--Wounds and injuries--Handbooks, manuals, etc.  I. Rohde, Rachel S., 1973- II. Title.
   [DNLM: 1. Hand Injuries--therapy--Handbooks.  WE 39 W422a 2009]
   RD559.W42 2009
   617.5'75044--dc22
                              2008039728

For permission to reprint material in another publication, contact SLACK Incorporated. Authorization to photocopy items for internal, personal, or academic use is granted by SLACK Incorporated provided that the appropriate fee is paid directly to Copyright Clearance Center. Prior to photocopying items, please contact the Copyright Clearance Center at 222 Rosewood Drive, Danvers, MA 01923 USA; phone: 978-750-8400; website: www.copyright.com; email: info@copyright.com

Printed in the United States of America.

Last digit is print number: 10   9   8   7   6   5   4   3   2   1

# Dedication

Over the course of almost four decades as a hand surgeon, I have had the good fortune of being nurtured by outstanding mentors and constantly stimulated by residents and fellows as an attending ortho-pedic surgeon. The enthusiasm, work ethic, and intellectual curiosity that residents and fellows possess have never ceased to amaze me. Their goal is to accumulate knowledge to achieve better results for patients with hand and upper extremity injuries.

The motivation for this book has come from them. They felt that a text dealing with acute management of hand injuries would serve as a reference for primary care physicians and emergency room physi-cians, thereby making them more knowledgeable in providing opti-mal treatment in the acute care setting.

I dedicate this work to the residents and fellows that I have been fortunate to work with throughout my career.

*Andrew J. Weiland, MD*

To my mentors who shared and continue to share their wisdom and enthusiasm for this special field, and granted me the opportunity to help and teach others...

To my colleagues who share the challenging task of taking care of people in this changing health care environment...

To my residents and students—now and always—whose eager-ness to learn reminds me both of my past, and the brightness of the future...

To my patients who entrust me to restore function and relieve pain, and who at the end of the day are the reason that I love what I do...

And last, but certainly not least, to my parents, who always have encouraged me to pursue my dreams...thank you.

*Rachel S. Rohde, MD*

# Contents

# Acknowledgments

The idea for this book came during our time together as mentor and fellow in training. At that time, it was just an idea that arose from wondering how people without hand training could be on the "front lines" temporizing these issues comfortably. There are many people who made it possible for this idea to become a reality.

Emily Altman, Kris Moonan, and Aviva Wolff are Certified Hand Therapists who fabricated and provided many of the splints depicted in Appendix A. They and their colleagues are indispensable members of our treatment teams, and we thank them for their contributions.

We also have had the pleasure of working with a terrific team at SLACK Incorporated. We would like to thank Carrie Kotlar, our acquisitions editor, who understood and shared our vision, and believed this to be as necessary a project as we did. We are grateful to Debra Steckel, our project editor, and Debra Toulson, our managing editor, as well as the artists at SLACK Incorporated for creating this work from a concept and dozens of computer files. They and their colleagues have made this work possible.

## About the Authors

Dr. Andrew J. Weiland is an attending orthopedic surgeon at the Hospital for Special Surgery. He is currently professor of Orthopedic Surgery and professor of Surgery (Plastic) at the Weill Medical College of Cornell University in New York. Dr. Weiland is the past president of the American Society for Reconstructive Microsurgery (1991), the American Society for Surgery of the Hand (1995), the American Orthopaedic Association (1998-1999), and the American Board of Orthopaedic Surgery (1998-1999), and treasurer of the American Academy of Orthopaedic Surgeons (2000-2003).

Dr. Rachel S. Rohde is a board certified attending orthopedic surgeon at William Beaumont Hospital in Royal Oak, Michigan. She completed her bachelor of science at the University of Michigan with highest distinction, following which she earned her doctorate of medicine from Harvard Medical School and Massachusetts Institute of Technology Division of Health Sciences and Technology. She trained in orthopedic surgery at the University of Pittsburgh and then completed fellowship training in hand and microvascular surgery at the Hospital for Special Surgery in New York City.

# Preface

Orthopedic conditions are among the most commonly evaluated complaints in the emergent and urgent care settings, as well as in primary care. In 2003, these musculoskeletal complaints accounted for the second highest number of physician visits in the United States. Many are acute problems involving the hand or wrist, an area of complex anatomy and function. Often, patients are evaluated by health care providers who might not have had the exposure or training to assess and manage certain complaints appropriately with confidence.

This book is written for physicians, physician assistants, nurse practitioners, resident physicians, and students who provide care in emergency room, urgent care, and primary practice settings, as well as for orthopedic surgeons who are not hand specialists. It is intended to be a concise, basic reference for the non-hand specialist to aid in the initial management of acute hand complaints. Although there is no text that can substitute for the advice of an experienced hand specialist, we hope that the following chapters will offer some guidance until that is available.

# Foreword

*Acute Management of Hand Injuries* is designed as an easy-to-use, quick reference guide for physicians treating acute hand and wrist conditions. The emergency room physician, primary care physician, student, nurse, physician's assistant and others who have not had formal hand surgery training will find this convenient, clearly written, and well-illustrated text a valuable asset. As an addition to its logical approach to the evaluation, the initial exam, and the definitive treatment of acute conditions, the authors provide some very innovative and attractive features that enhance the text's value. In a group of well-constructed appendices, the authors describe common techniques such as the performance of digital blocks and the fabrication and application of commonly needed splints. Others describe currently recommended antibiotic treatment for felons, paronychia, and suppurative flexor tenosynovitis, and reference checks for tetanus and rabies immunization. Another useful feature is the frequent use of illustrative cases that demonstrate, for instance, the key to effective evaluation of the patient with a wrist injury, with anatomical snuffbox tenderness, and with suspected scaphoid fracture. Located at the end of each chapter is a short list of well-selected and timely references on the subject.

The authors are to be congratulated on delivering such an effective guide to the principles and practice of emergency hand and wrist diagnosis and treatment. The book will prove to be an invaluable addition to the libraries, and to the pockets, of those who are on the front line, where initial management is so critical to the final outcome.

*Richard H. Gelberman, MD*
*Professor and Chairman*
*Department of Orthopedic Surgery*
*Washington University School of Medicine*

# Introduction

This book is written and organized for use by health care providers who provide care for patients with urgent hand and wrist complaints in the emergency room, urgent care, and other practice settings.

The first chapter is an introduction to evaluating these conditions, including detailed pictures illustrating a hand examination. The chapters that follow are divided into sections detailing the mechanisms of injury, evaluation, initial treatment, definitive treatment, and potential problems encountered in the most common hand complaints. At the end of each section, we suggest readings that we think are appropriate for further education regarding each subject.

Appendices illustrate techniques such as splinting, administering digital anesthesia, and removing tight rings as well as provide quick references regarding orthopedic abbreviations and tetanus protocols.

This text is not intended to replace appropriate supervision by, or consultation of, providers with more experience treating hand and wrist injuries, but rather to serve as a quick reference to guide acute care and early, appropriate referral for definitive management.

# Section I

## Assessment of Acute Hand Injury Patients: The Basics

# chapter 1

# EVALUATING PATIENTS WITH URGENT HAND INJURIES

Performing a history and physical examination on a patient who presents with an acute hand injury is a skill that is refined with experience. It takes many years of training to be an expert in this area, so do not feel discouraged if you find yourself in unfamiliar territory. What follows are some basic principles to help keep you on the right track.

***Ask the Important Questions.*** The first 3 things you want to know about anyone presenting with a hand injury are age, hand dominance, and occupation. These significant characteristics are important factors that affect treatment options and outcomes.

- **Age** can work for or against a patient in terms of recovery. For example, we know that nerve repairs tend to be more successful in younger patients than older patients. However, we also know that joint surfaces affected by fractures can go on to develop arthritis over time; this might not lead to problems in the wrist of an 82 year old, but certainly might in a 28 year old.

- **Hand dominance** will give you and the patient an idea of how much this will affect him or her acutely and in the future. Even the simplest daily activities, such as brushing one's teeth, become more difficult when using the nondominant hand.

- **Occupation** also is important in determining what effect an injury will have on this patient's future. For example, a bad wrist fracture in a massage therapist might result in more significant impairment than the same fracture in someone who works primarily at a desk. A laborer who has a digital amputation might be better served with a revision and closure of the amputation stump than by replantation of the digit because he or she likely would be less symptomatic and be able to return to work sooner.

- **Medical comorbidities** can be causative or contributing factors. Diabetes can be associated with hand conditions ranging from trigger finger to cellulitis; gout often is not recognized when it presents in the hand and wrist. Smoking (which we will call a "comorbidity") impairs blood flow and can inhibit healing of bone and soft tissues. Knowing that such conditions can be associated with hand complaints will help you diagnose and treat.

***Get the Details***. It sometimes is difficult to listen to the stories of hand injuries, but it is extremely important to find out what happened, where, when, and why. A laceration by a clean kitchen knife is not as concerning as one by a dirty lawnmower blade; a puncture wound by a thorn is not as emergent as one by a tooth (see Chapter 30). An infection that has developed over a few days is different from one that becomes raging within hours. Ask the patient or witnesses for the details and make sure that you have a clear understanding of what happened.

***Do a Thorough Evaluation***. It is very important to perform an accurate assessment of the extremity. Use the basic principles: inspection, palpation, range of motion, sensory examination, vascular examination, strength testing. It helps to draw a diagram of the injured area and label any lacerations, deformities, deficits, etc. so that you can remember and document the status at that time. Draw and label both dorsal and volar (palmar) views, and label the side (right versus left) and the digit, if applicable. A diagram template can be found in Appendix I. Also, remember to check for other injuries; often the most apparent is the one that is diagnosed, but pay close attention to injuries that can be missed (Figure 1-1). The examination will be covered in more detail in the next chapter.

***Get the Right Studies***. Always get a set of radiographs even if you do not suspect a fracture. A full set of radiographs (usually 3 views) is necessary in the hand and wrist. In addition to showing fractures and dislocations, radiographs can show foreign bodies, air, soft tissue swelling, and other important characteristics that are helpful for treatment now and later. Make sure you look at all studies that you order, rather than relying on someone's reading; you might pick up something that he or she missed.

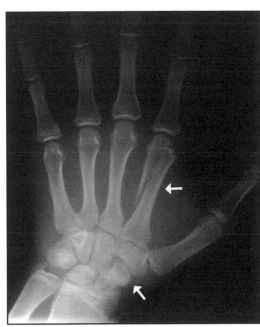

**Figure 1-1.** This 17-year-old right-hand dominant quarterback fell during a game and sustained an injury to his index metacarpal. The initial provider did not see the scaphoid fracture at the edge of the film, a fracture that likely had been missed by another provider whom the patient had seen 3 years before the recent injury.

***Manage Expectations.*** Patients often will ask you what they can expect in the near and far future. Each chapter of this book includes an anticipated definitive treatment plan to help guide you in answering these questions. However, it is helpful to explain to patients that every person and every injury has a different healing potential, so much of what happens next will depend on those differences. It is acceptable to tell them that you are not the hand specialist and that you do not know all the answers; after all, your hand specialist likely would not answer the questions about most of the non-hand conditions you treat, and honesty is always best.

***Ask for Help.*** If you are uncertain about how to manage something, ask. Ask a colleague, a supervisor, a consultant, someone who has more experience than you. It is a good idea to establish a relationship with one or more hand specialists in your area whom you feel comfortable contacting for advice. In the hospital setting, there usually is a hand surgeon on call who might be able to help you by phone or in person. It is better for everyone if you ask for help before you do something about which you are unsure.

***Refer Early.*** Patients never complain that they wish they had not seen a hand specialist so early, and they never are upset when a hand specialist gives them good news (eg, "it is unlikely that this is a fracture"). The bad news—when it has to come—is unavoidable, but it is the late bad news that is a problem. Most acute conditions should be referred as soon as possible (within a few days) so that the diagnosis can be confirmed, and a definitive treatment plan can be made.

These are just a few pearls to keep in mind as you treat patients with acute hand complaints. Helping these people can be very gratifying; you truly are a part of each patient's road to recovery.

chapter *2*

# EXAMINATION OF THE HAND

The complex anatomy of the hand is beyond the focus of this book, but understanding the anatomy is key to performing a thorough, accurate examination, and facilitating a proper diagnosis and course of management. Documentation and communication of examination findings are easier when descriptive terms referring to surface anatomy (Figure 2-1) and underlying bone and joint architecture are used.

*Inspect* the hand for skin lacerations, edema, ecchymosis, and deformity. These often are indicative of a serious injury.

*Palpate* for tenderness, crepitation, fluctuant areas, and instability.

*Assess the range of motion* of the elbow—flexion/extension; the forearm—pronation/supination; the wrist—flexion/extension and radial/ulnar deviation; and the digits—flexion/extension of the metacarpophalangeal joints (MPJ), the proximal interphalangeal joints (PIPJ), the distal interphalangeal joints (DIPJ), and adduction/abduction of thumb at the carpal metacarpal joints (CMCJ).

*Examine the function and motor strength* of muscles and tendons (Figures 2-2A-E, 2-3A-E, 2-4A-E). For communication and comparison purposes, motor strength can be graded on a scale from 0 to 5:

| | |
|---|---|
| 0/5 | No detectable muscle function |
| 1/5 | Muscle visibly contracts or "flickers" |
| 2/5 | Muscle functions with gravity eliminated |
| 3/5 | Muscle functions against gravity, but not against any other resistance |
| 4/5 | Muscle functions against examiner's resistance, but not at full strength |
| 5/5 | Muscle functions against examiner's full resistance ("normal"). |

*Evaluate sensation* using a 2-point discrimination. This can be performed using a caliper (Figure 2-5) or a paper clip. A sensory deficit is indicated by the inability to discriminate 2 points as little as 6 mm apart. This should be documented in all nerve distributions:

7

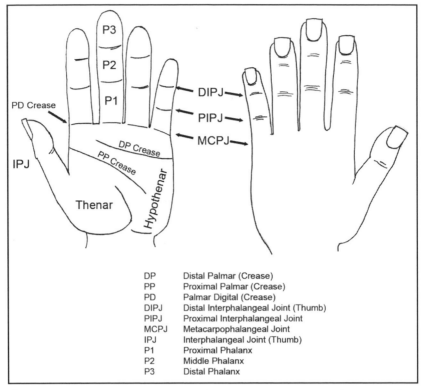

| | |
|---|---|
| DP | Distal Palmar (Crease) |
| PP | Proximal Palmar (Crease) |
| PD | Palmar Digital (Crease) |
| DIPJ | Distal Interphalangeal Joint (Thumb) |
| PIPJ | Proximal Interphalangeal Joint |
| MCPJ | Metacarpophalangeal Joint |
| IPJ | Interphalangeal Joint (Thumb) |
| P1 | Proximal Phalanx |
| P2 | Middle Phalanx |
| P3 | Distal Phalanx |

**Figure 2-1.** Surface anatomy can be used to describe locations of tenderness, swelling, lacerations, and deformities.

median, ulnar, and radial (Figure 2-6), and in the radial and ulnar digital nerve distributions of each digit.

*Assess perfusion* using skin color, nail bed blanching, digital Doppler examination, and Allen's test. To perform Allen's test at the wrist:

- Place slight manual pressure on the patient's radial and ulnar arteries at the wrist.

- Ask the patient to make a fist and extend the digit multiple times to exsanguinate (remove blood from) the hand, then occlude the radial and ulnar arteries.

- Release pressure on the radial artery while maintaining occlusion of the ulnar artery; perfusion of the hand within 5 seconds indicates a patent radial artery and circulation through the arch to the hand.

- Repeat the examination, releasing the ulnar artery occlusion and maintaining pressure on the radial artery to assess patency of the ulnar artery and perfusion through the arch.

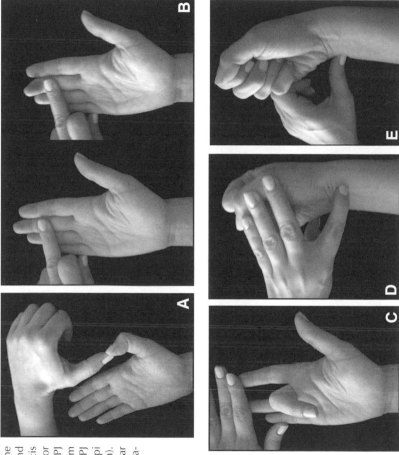

**Figures 2-2A-E.** Testing of the "extrinsic flexors" of the hand and wrist. (A) Flexor pollicis longus (IPJ flexion). (B) Flexor digitorum profundus (DIPJ flexion). (C) Flexor digitorum superficialis (isolated PIPJ flexion). (D) Flexor carpi radialis (radial wrist flexion). (E) Flexor carpi ulnaris (ulnar wrist flexion/ulnar wrist deviation).

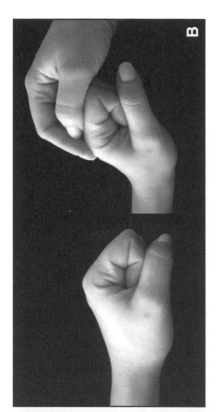

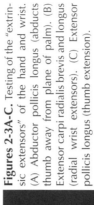

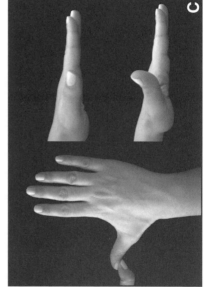

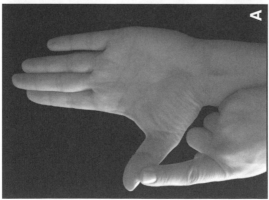

**Figures 2-3A-C.** Testing of the "extrinsic extensors" of the hand and wrist. (A) Abductor pollicis longus (abducts thumb away from plane of palm). (B) Extensor carpi radialis brevis and longus (radial wrist extensors). (C) Extensor pollicis longus (thumb extension).

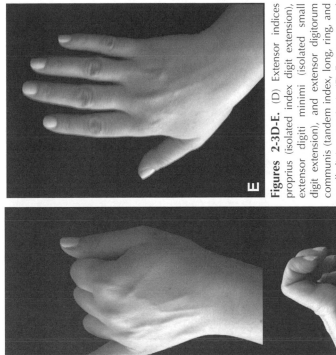

**Figures 2-3D-E.** (D) Extensor indices proprius (isolated index digit extension), extensor digiti minimi (isolated small digit extension), and extensor digitorum communis (tandem index, long, ring, and small digit extension). (E) Extensor carpi ulnaris (ulnar wrist extension/deviation).

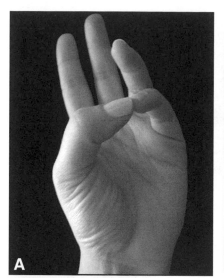

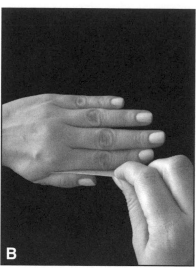

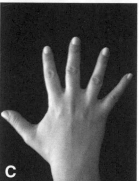

**Figures 2-4A-E.** Testing of major "intrinsic" muscles of the hand. (A) Opponens pollicis (opposition of thumb to small finger). (B) First dorsal interosseous (thumb adduction). (C) Interossei (abduction and adduction of digits). (D) Abductor digiti minimi (abduction of small digit). Froment's sign (E) is "positive" when instead of using the first dorsal interosseous to grasp a piece of paper (as in B), the patient flexes the IPJ of the thumb; this is indicative of an ulnar nerve injury, in which case the median-innervated flexor pollicis longus (FPL) is used instead of the ulnar-innervated adductors.

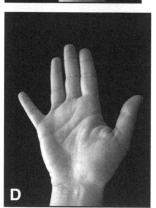

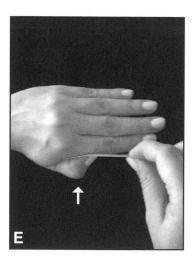

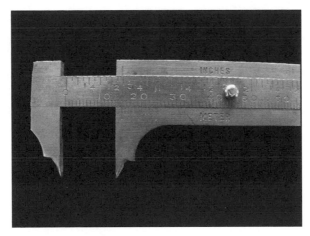

**Figure 2-5.** This caliper was machined to enable measurement of 2-point discrimination.

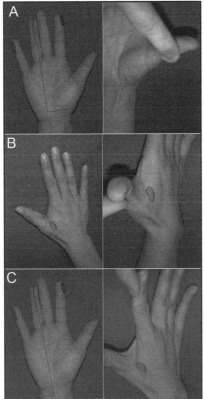

**Figure 2-6.** "Quick tests" to evaluate function of median, radial, and ulnar nerves in the hand. The median nerve (A) generally provides sensation to the thumb, index, and long fingers, and radial half of the ring finger; testing thumb abduction (away from the plane of the palm) assesses median-innervated thenar musculature (ask the patient to keep the back of his or her hand on the table and lift his or her thumb toward the ceiling). The radial nerve (B) provides sensation on the dorsum of the first web space and can be tested grossly by checking resisted thumb extension, an action of the extensor pollicis longus (ask the patient to lift his or her thumb up like he or she is trying to hitch a ride). The ulnar nerve (C) innervates the small finger and ulnar half of the ring finger; gross testing of ulnar motor function includes interosseous testing (ask the patient to spread his or her fingers apart and hold them there).

# Section II

## Bone and Joint Injuries

# chapter 3

# GENERAL CONCEPTS: "DO I NEED SURGERY?"

Fractures and dislocations of the hand and wrist are very common. Patients understandably will have questions regarding the "next step" in their care. Although you certainly cannot be expected to have all the answers, it is helpful for a nonspecialist to have a basic understanding of what likely will, or will not, need operative intervention. In general, fractures and dislocations that likely will need intervention include (but are not limited to):

- **Open injuries**: Like open fractures in other areas of the body, those in the hand and wrist require irrigation and debridement to prevent infection. This is especially true for contaminated wounds. Open injuries also can be associated with nerve, tendon, and vessel injuries that might need to be addressed. Fortunately, the hand has a better blood supply than most areas, and most open fractures without gross contamination can be irrigated in the urgent care setting and scheduled for elective surgery within a few days.

- **Malrotation or "scissoring"** of the digits is unacceptable. This is identified by asking the patient to try to make a fist slowly, and looking at the volar aspect of the hand. Despite the pain and swelling, patients usually can show you whether they have overlapping digits with fist formation. Any overlap is an indication for reduction (at least), with possible fixation.

- **Severe crush injuries** can be associated with compartment syndrome. Even if no fractures are identified, pressures can build high enough that fasciotomies, or release of the fascia (and thus, release of pressure), are required.

- **Multiple metacarpal fractures** might need operative fixation to maintain stability.

- **Dislocations** that cannot be reduced without surgery will need relatively urgent operative treatment to prevent further soft tissue and cartilage damage.

- **Inherently unstable fracture patterns** might be difficult to recognize for a nonspecialist. A common example is the long oblique or spiral fracture of the phalanx (Figure 3-1). Because of the complex pulls of the tendon mechanisms about the digit, these tend to shorten and displace if not fixed.

- **Displaced fractures that extend into a joint surface** usually need to be addressed operatively to ensure that the joint surface is restored properly to avoid arthritis and pain in the future. Major exceptions to this are the mallet fracture from the dorsum of the distal phalanx, and the volar plate avulsion fracture from the middle phalanx with a proximal interphalangeal (PIP) joint dislocation; you will see in the upcoming chapters that these usually can be treated without surgery.

- **Displaced scaphoid fractures** need to be reduced and fixed operatively to prevent the scaphoid from dying (avascular necrosis) and to prevent the development of wrist arthritis.

Although this list is not all-inclusive, it can be used as a general guide to manage the expectations of patients you will see. Remember, if you do not know the answer, just be honest with the patient and make an early referral; again, it would be difficult to find a patient who is upset for having been referred to a specialist too early.

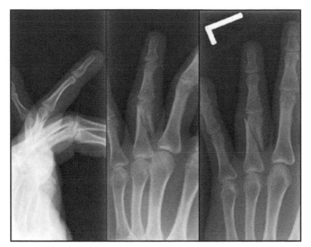

**Figure 3-1.** This 28-year-old right-hand-dominant female realtor sustained a forceful "twisting" (rotational) injury of her left ring finger. She presented to the office 8 days later, at which time clinical evaluation revealed a stiff, swollen digit but malrotation could not be assessed because of significant edema. Radiographs show this long oblique spiral fracture of the proximal phalanx with shortening. This is an example of an unstable fracture pattern which likely will continue to displace proximally and rotate. This is an example of a fracture that requires operative treatment.

# chapter 4

# MALLET FRACTURES

"Mallet fracture," or Type IV mallet finger, is an avulsion fracture of the distal phalanx by the extensor tendon. This may or may not lead to joint subluxation, which must be identified and corrected as soon as possible.

## Mechanism of Injury

- Forced extension of the distal phalanx against resistance causes the extensor tendon to avulse a small piece of dorsal distal phalanx.
- This is common in sports when a ball hits the dorsum of the fingertip, sometimes called "baseball finger."

## Evaluation

- The patient usually presents complaining of an inability to straighten a finger. The patient might have noticed this condition weeks or months ago and thought it would go away, but it did not.
- The digit rests with the distal interphalangeal (DIP) joint in flexion (Figure 4-1). If this is "chronic" (>4 weeks), the digit might rest in a "swan neck" deformity, with the DIP joint in flexion and the PIP joint in hyperextension.
- When asked, the patient is unable to extend actively at the DIP joint.
- Radiographs reveal an avulsion fragment of the dorsal distal phalanx (Figure 4-2), and sometimes can show subluxation of the joint.

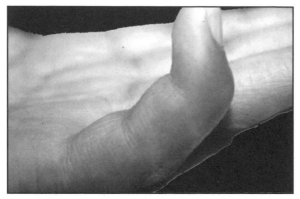

**Figure 4-1.** Mallet finger deformity.

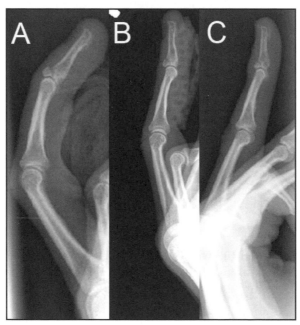

**Figure 4-2.** Lateral radiographs of a digit showing displaced mallet fracture (A), excellent alignment of the joint after reduction of the fracture using DIP hyperextension splint (B), and healing at 8 weeks with full active extension and a congruent joint (C).

- This also is referred to as a "bony mallet" because of the involved bone fragment, distinguishing it from a simple "mallet" in which only the extensor tendon is avulsed (see Chapter 17).

## Acute Treatment

- Splint the DIP joint in slight hyperextension (see Figure 4-2B; also see Appendix A, Figure A-1). If a "Stax" finger splint is available, it can be applied. An aluminum/foam splint can be used temporarily as well, molding the splint so that the DIP joint is slightly hyperextended and the PIP joint is free to move. Too much hyperextension at the DIP joint can decrease the blood supply there and lead to skin problems.
- Inform the patient that the splint needs to stay on all the time until the hand is seen by a specialist. Instruct the patient that the splint needs to be worn for 6 to 8 weeks, and if the splint is removed and the joint is allowed to flex even slightly, the tendon can tear again and the "clock" resets to zero.
- Repeat radiographs of the joint with the hyperextension splint in place; the alignment might not be perfect (the mallet fracture rarely reduces completely), but the joint should be congruent, not subluxated (Figure 4-3).

## Definitive Treatment (Refer to Hand Specialist)

- Acute mallet fractures usually can be treated closed in a DIP hyperextension splint for 6 to 8 weeks. Certified hand therapists generally are very skilled at making splints that fit more comfortably than the "one size fits all" splints.
- Patients are instructed regarding how to care for their skin during the extended period of immobilization.
- Joint subluxation is an indication for surgery, which might include reduction of the joint and percutaneous pin fixation until healing occurs.
- Patients are checked periodically, both clinically and radiographically, for alignment and healing (see Figure 4-2C).
- Mallet finger without fracture (tendon avulsion only) is treated for 6 to 8 weeks with a hyperextension splint (see Chapter 17).

## Potential Problems

- DIP hyperextension splints are cumbersome and patients often

**Figure 4-3.** This mallet finger involves joint subluxation. Attempted reduction using slight DIP joint hyperextension did not result in a congruent joint (right). This injury subsequently was treated operatively to maintain joint alignment.

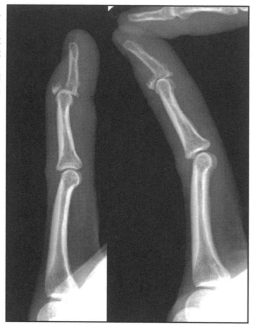

remove them; removal and allowance of the joint to flex resets the 6- to 8-week clock back to zero.

- Skin breakdown can be an issue with splinting; this often can be attributed to too much hyperextension.
- Nail deformity is a rare but reported potential complication.
- If addressed (or readdressed) late (>4 weeks), a mallet injury can be considered "chronic." Chronic injuries might not heal without surgery, either reparative or reconstructive. Patients who undergo surgical treatment for a mallet injury have an increased risk of infection, nail deformities, hardware problems, pain, and other complications.
- Erythema and swelling just proximal to the base of the nail can persist for several months.

## Suggested Reading

Bendre AA, Hartigan BJ, Kalainov DM. Mallet finger. *J Am Acad Orthop Surg.* 2005;13(5):336-344.

Tuttle HG, Olvey SP, Stern PJ. Tendon avulsion injuries of the distal phalanx. *Clin Orthop Rel Res.* 2006;445:157-168.

# chapter 5

# FINGERTIP INJURIES: DISTAL PHALANX FRACTURES AND NAIL BED LACERATIONS

Fingertip injuries are extremely common. Treatment of many of these can be accomplished by an experienced provider in an urgent or emergent care setting. Proper lighting and equipment are essential to evaluate the characteristics of the injury and manage appropriately.

## Mechanism of Injury

- Crush injuries and power equipment (table saw, snow blowers, lawnmowers) are common causes of distal phalanx fractures.
- Clean lacerations (knife or other sharp object) can create nail bed injury without phalanx fracture.
- The nail bed is adherent to the distal phalanx periosteum, so the nail bed is injured by definition with a distal phalanx fracture.

## Evaluation

- Evaluate level and direction of injury: transverse, volar oblique, dorsal oblique (Figure 5-1).
- Assess and diagram areas of laceration, skin loss, and direction of distal amputation (if present).
- Determine the extent of soft tissue loss, and whether there is exposed bone.
- Closed injuries may present with a subungual hematoma, or a dark discoloration and pressure beneath the nail plate.

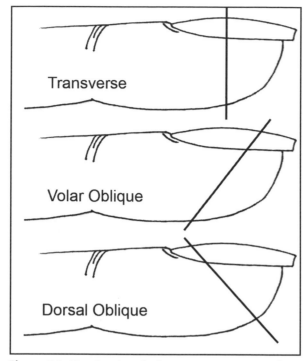

**Figure 5-1.** The direction of a fingertip amputation can determine treatment options; descriptive terms include transverse (top), volar or palmar oblique (middle), and dorsal oblique (bottom).

- Open injuries usually demonstrate either a simple laceration through the skin, or a laceration through the nail plate and underlying nail bed.
- Document sensory and perfusion examination.
- Radiographs will demonstrate to what degree the bone fragments are comminuted or displaced, and the presence of any radiopaque foreign material (Figure 5-2).

## Acute Treatment

- Tetanus should be administered if indicated (Appendix C), as well as antibiotics if a fracture is present (a nail bed injury technically is an open fracture).

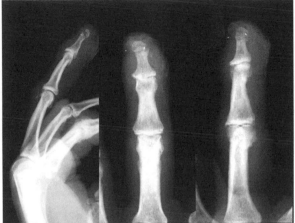

**Figure 5-2.** Lateral, anterior-posterior (AP), and oblique radiograph showing a distal phalanx tuft fracture following a band saw injury. A tuft fracture in a closed injury also is indicative of injury to the nail bed.

- Sterile preparation and draping of the entire hand comfortably positioned on a Mayo (or other bedside) table allows space and support, enabling the procedure to be performed comfortably and sterilely.

- A digital block can be used to provide anesthesia (Appendix B).

- Irrigation of the wound with saline will help decrease the risk of infection and enable you to evaluate the injury better.

- If the skin edges can be aligned well without tension, skin can be sutured with 5-0 nylon suture in adolescents and adults. An absorbable suture (such as chromic or plain) can be used in children so that suture removal (which can be traumatic) will not be necessary.

- In cases of tip amputation without exposed bone, healing by secondary intention is recommended. Irrigation of the wound is followed by application of a nonadherent dressing and referral to a hand surgeon.

- If a subungual hematoma does not involve more than 50% of the nail plate, simple decompression using an 18-gauge needle will relieve the pressure, and is an acceptable method of treatment. If the hematoma involves more than 50% of the nail plate, the nail should be removed and the sterile matrix repaired with 6-0 chromic suture (Figure 5-3).

- Nail bed repair:
  - Remove the nail plate carefully (a hemostat or Freer elevator placed under the nail plate can be used); save the nail plate as you will need it later.

**Figure 5-3.** This crush injury resulted in a distal phalanx fracture with considerable subungual hematoma. Removal of the nail plate revealed a large nail bed laceration. This was repaired with 6-0 chromic suture. The nail plate was replaced under the eponychial fold; if the nail plate is not available, foil (such as from a suture package) may be inserted instead. *For a full-color version, see page CA-I of the Color Atlas.*

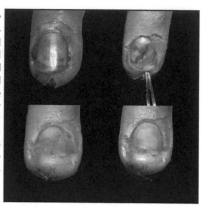

♦ Repair the nail bed as anatomically as possible using 6-0 absorbable (plain or chromic) suture.

♦ Examine the "back" of the nail plate for remnants of the nail bed; these can be removed from the nail plate and sutured in place. If much of the sterile matrix is absent, the patient might require a nail bed graft by a hand surgeon.

♦ Following repair of the nail bed, create a "hole" in the nail plate using a sharp blade or 18-gauge needle. Replace the nail plate beneath the eponychial fold and suture the plate in place with nylon suture (Figure 5-4).

♦ If the nail plate is unavailable, aluminum foil can be used to create a nail plate to prevent the eponychial fold from scarring. Failure to keep the eponychial fold open can result in nail deformity or pain as the nail "tries" to grow.

♦ Dress the wound with nonadherent dressing, sterile gauze, and a simple splint.

• Refer fingertip injuries for early evaluation by a hand surgeon. The patient does not need to do any dressing changes until he or she is seen by the specialist.

## Definitive Treatment (Refer to Hand Specialist)

• Tip amputations without exposed bone heal well by secondary intention. Daily soaks in dilute hydrogen peroxide (50% hydro-

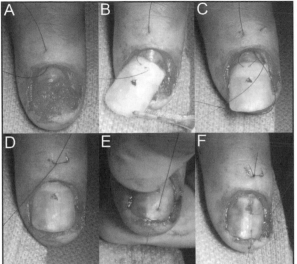

**Figure 5-4.** The nail plate is replaced beneath the eponychial fold and sutured as shown with 5-0 nylon to prevent dislodgement (A-D). An additional suture through the nail plate into the hyponychium (E-F) secures the plate to the nail bed. Note drainage hole placed in nail plate with blade. *For a full-color version, see page CA-I of the Color Atlas.*

gen peroxide and 50% sterile water) and dressing changes allow healing over a period of several weeks. Patients are encouraged to perform range of motion exercises and edema control, consulting a hand therapist if necessary. Formal desensitization instruction may be used following healing.

- Tip amputations with exposed bone may require shortening, skin grafting, or other procedures depending on the level and direction of amputation.

- Proper repair of a nail bed injury is essential. If it can be completed well in your health care setting (primarily emergency room), and if you are comfortable with this skill, great. If not, the patient should be seen by a hand specialist as soon as possible to treat this appropriately.

- Following proper repair, patients generally have skin sutures removed (remember, nail bed sutures are absorbable) and begin range of motion exercises when the wound has healed.

## Potential Problems

- Nail deformity is an issue even in the best situation. Patients need to be told (and reminded) that the nail likely will never be the same again. Painful or unsightly nail deformities can develop that might be treated surgically.

• Crush and avulsion injuries at the fingertip can result in cold intolerance or other hypersensitivity.

• Infections occur because many of these injuries occur in contaminated settings.

## SUGGESTED READING

Ashbell TS, Kleinert HE, Putcha SM, Kutz JE. The deformed finger nail, a frequent result of failure to repair nail bed injuries. *J Trauma.* 1967;7(2):177-190.

Brown RE. Acute nail bed injuries. *Hand Clin.* 2002;18(4):561-575.

Fassler PR. Fingertip injuries: evaluation and treatment. *J Am Acad Orthop Surg.* 1996;4:84-92.

Martin C, González del Pino J. Controversies in the treatment of fingertip amputations. Conservative versus surgical reconstruction. *Clin Orthop Relat Res.* 1998;353:63-73.

Stevenson TR. Fingertip and nailbed injuries. *Orthop Clin North Am.* 1992;23(1): 149-159.

Zook EG, Guy RJ, Russell RC. A study of nail bed injuries: causes, treatment, and prognosis. *J Hand Surg.* 1984;9A(2):247-252.

# chapter 6

# MIDDLE AND PROXIMAL PHALANX FRACTURES

There is a common misconception that nothing is done for "finger fractures." However, finger fractures range from nondisplaced extra-articular fractures to those that involve significant comminution, displacement, or joint disruption. Many of these need to be addressed early to prevent stiffness or improper healing. Patients should be reminded of the importance of follow-up appointments.

## Mechanism of Injury

- Twisting, bending, direct blow, or crushing forces can fracture the middle and proximal phalanges.
- The mechanism of injury will determine the fracture configuration:
  - Twisting/torsion force results in a spiral fracture
  - Bending or direct blow results in a transverse or oblique fracture
  - Crushing results in a comminuted fracture

## Evaluation

- Patients will complain of pain, swelling, or loss of motion following trauma.
- Edema, ecchymosis, and tenderness are common.
- Look for open injuries, which predispose to infection.
- Examine for malrotation or "scissoring/overlap" of digits with slow, gentle fist formation.

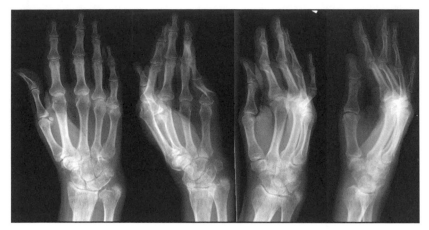

**Figure 6-1.** This patient presented with pain and deformity at the base of her right small finger. Radiographs show a proximal phalanx fracture; the apex volar angulation is appreciated best on the lateral views.

- AP, lateral, and oblique radiographs of all questionable areas should be obtained and reviewed (Figure 6-1). Look closely at the lateral radiograph, which is difficult to evaluate, but might be the only view that shows displacement or angulation of a phalanx fracture.

## Acute Treatment

- If there is gross deformity, and you are comfortable with performing closed reduction of fractures, attempt a closed reduction to align fracture fragments better. Closed reductions generally involve accentuation of the deformity, gentle traction, and correction of the deformity.
- Place the hand in a well-padded plaster volar splint or ulnar gutter splint for comfort and immobilization.
- Repeat radiographs and reevaluate after any fracture manipulation.
- Advise the patient not to bear weight on the injured hand, apply ice, and elevate above the level of the heart to minimize swelling.

## Definitive Treatment (Refer to Hand Specialist)

- Malrotation/scissoring with digit flexion, unstable fracture pattern, displacement, and intra-articular extension are indicators for reduction and possible fixation; these should be seen by a hand surgeon within a few days. Fractures that have been reduced also should be reevaluated early because loss of reduction is common, especially as edema resolves.
- Fractures able to be treated nonoperatively are treated with immobilization until some healing has occurred, followed by protected range of motion.
- These fractures usually take 3 to 6 weeks to heal.

## Potential Problems

- Malunion (or healing in the wrong position) or finger stiffness can result if not treated appropriately and expeditiously.
- Arthritic pain can occur in the future if the fracture extends into the joint surface.

*SUGGESTED READING*

Kozin SH, Thoder JJ, Lieberman G. Operative treatment of metacarpal and phalangeal shaft fractures. *J Am Acad Orthop Surg.* 2000;8(2):111-121.

Lee SG, Jupiter JB. Phalangeal and metacarpal fractures of the hand. *Hand Clin.* 2000;16(3):323-332.

# chapter 7

# PROXIMAL INTERPHALANGEAL JOINT DISLOCATIONS AND VOLAR PLATE INJURIES

The PIP joint normally has the largest arc of motion of the three joints in the digit, but also is the most likely to develop stiffness. A seemingly simple "jammed finger" can become stiff and hinder grip. Early stabilization and guided motion are needed to ensure a good outcome.

## Mechanism of Injury

- Patients describe "jamming" or "catching" of the finger, particularly while playing sports. This force results in hyperextension and rotation at the PIP joint, dislocating the joint, usually with tearing of the radial collateral ligament.
- Patients might report that the finger was out of joint, but they pulled it back into place.
- Hyperextension injuries also can result in tearing of the volar plate, an area of soft tissue on the palmar aspect of the PIP joint.

## Evaluation

- Inspect for deformity, swelling, and ecchymosis.
- Palpate for tenderness, especially along the volar plate (palmar to the PIP joint) and collateral ligaments (on the sides of the PIP joint).
- AP, oblique, and true lateral radiographs are needed to assess congruency of the joint surface and presence of fracture.

**Figure 7-1.** (A) PIP joint fracture-dislocation shows dorsal subluxation of the middle phalanx following attempted reduction. (B) A dorsal block splint was applied with the PIP joint flexed approximately 45°, and repeat lateral radiograph demonstrated alignment of the joint with reduction of the avulsion fracture. The degree of splint flexion was reduced (ie, the splint was extended) gradually over the next several weeks, and motion of the digit was maintained. (C) Radiographs at 6 weeks showed healing with concentric alignment of the joint.

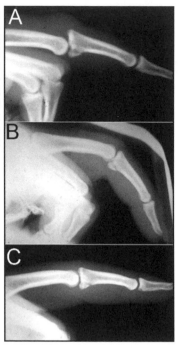

## Acute Treatment

- If the joint is dislocated, gentle increased hyperextension, traction, and pressure on the dorsum of the middle phalanx generally will allow reduction.

- Always take postreduction radiographs to ensure that the joint is aligned congruently.

- Stability can be tested by true lateral radiograph with the digit in full extension; if a joint is unstable because of soft tissue damage, this extension will cause the joint to subluxate or redislocate.

- Volar plate injuries without any radiographic evidence of injury still can cause significant swelling and stiffness; these can be treated with buddy taping and early range of motion exercises.

- Pure dislocations without fractures generally are stable and also can be treated with buddy taping for 6 weeks.

- Avulsion fractures can cause instability, especially if more than 20% of the joint surface is involved (Figure 7-1A). Apply dorsal blocking splint at approximately 30° and check reduction on lateral radiograph (Figure 7-1B).

## Definitive Treatment (Refer to Hand Specialist)

- If the joint is stable with buddy taping, it can be treated with buddy taping, early motion, and edema control. Hand therapy can be helpful if the patient needs some guidance or is hesitant to move the digit. Again, even a soft tissue injury at the volar plate without a fracture can cause significant problems if not addressed and mobilized.
- If the joint is stable with a dorsal blocking splint, early motion and edema control is initiated, and the splint is adjusted to extend gradually over the next 4 weeks, until the joint is stable in full extension.
- If the joint is inherently unstable (usually because of large fracture fragment or interposition of soft tissue within the joint) or the joint is not well-reduced with a dorsal blocking splint, it will require open reduction internal fixation (ORIF), pinning, external fixation, or other surgical procedures.

## Potential Problems

- Stiffness, pain, and arthritis can result if the joint is not reduced congruently or if the joint is immobilized for a prolonged period.
- Edema tends to persist for months to years.

*SUGGESTED READING*

Blazar PE, Steinberg DR. Fractures of the proximal interphalangeal joint. *J Am Acad Orthop Surg.* 2000;8(6):383-390.

Freiberg A, Pollard BA, Macdonald MR, Duncan MJ. Management of proximal interphalangeal joint injuries. *Hand Clin.* 2006;22(3):235-242.

# chapter 8

# GAMEKEEPER'S THUMB

The term "gamekeeper's thumb" was coined to describe the chronic ligament injury sustained by breaking the necks of game (rabbits) between the thumb and rest of the hand. Today, we also refer to it as "skier's thumb," as skiers often sustain this injury while holding the pole between the thumb and the index finger. It is for this reason that skiers are advised to toss the poles away if falling and not to loop them to their wrists; modern ski equipment thankfully has molded hand grips instead of wrist straps.

## Mechanism of Injury

- A radially (laterally) directed force at the metacarpophalangeal (MCP) joint of the thumb tears the ulnar collateral ligament (partially or completely) either from the metacarpal or, more commonly, the proximal phalanx (85%).

## Evaluation

- Patients can present complaining of pain at the ulnar aspect of the thumb MCP joint.
- Examination reveals swelling and ecchymosis at this area.
- The patient complains of pain, and the examiner notes instability, with radially directed stress at the MCP joint. Examine with the thumb fully extended, and with the thumb MCP at 30°. Compare to the unaffected hand to make sure that this is not symmetrical laxity.
- Radiographs sometimes reveal an avulsion fracture (Figure 8-1), but more often do not.

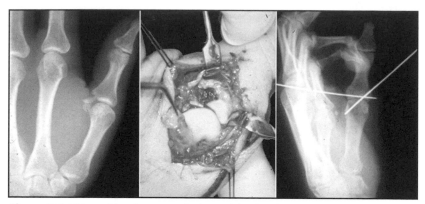

**Figure 8-1.** This avulsion fracture at the base of the thumb proximal phalanx is a type of "bony gamekeeper's thumb." Open reduction of the rotated fragment with fixation was necessary to restore stability and congruity of the joint.

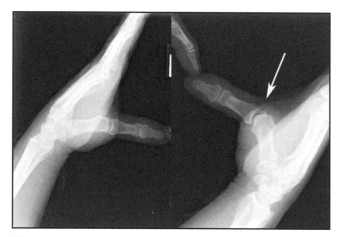

**Figure 8-2.** Stress radiographs can be used to determine whether the MCP joint of the thumb "opens" when a radially directed stress is applied. The image on the left demonstrates a stress view of the uninjured thumb MCP joint; the image on the right shows opening at the ulnar aspect of the MCP joint of the injured thumb, confirming ulnar collateral ligament injury.

- Stress radiographs can be used to ascertain opening of the joint space (Figure 8-2).

## Acute Treatment

- Apply a well-padded thumb spica splint to immobilize the MCP joint of thumb.
- Advise the patient to rest, use ice, and elevate.

## Definitive Treatment (Refer to Hand Specialist)

- Examination sometimes provides enough information to confirm the diagnosis; sometimes magnetic resonance imaging (MRI) is ordered (nonemergently) to look for Stener lesion— tissue interposed that will prevent ligament healing without surgical intervention.
- If there is a Stener lesion, the patient will need operative treatment.
- If there is no Stener lesion, the surgeon and patient will decide whether to treat this operatively with ligament repair, or nonoperatively with immobilization.

## Potential Problems

- If left untreated, this can lead to chronic instability, arthritis, as well as activity-related pain (even pain with writing).
- Treatment of chronic gamekeeper's thumb involves ulnar collateral ligament reconstruction or arthrodesis (fusion) of the MCP joint if it is arthritic.

*SUGGESTED READING*

Heim D. The skier's thumb. *Acta Orthop Belg.* 1999;65(4):440-446.
Morgan WJ, Slowman LS. Acute hand and wrist injuries in athletes: evaluation and management. *J Am Acad Orthop Surg.* 2001;9(6):389-400.

# chapter 9

# METACARPAL FRACTURES

Metacarpal fractures commonly result from a direct blow to the hand. Although many metacarpal fractures can be treated nonoperatively, intra-articular or displaced fractures might require reduction, with or without surgical fixation.

## Mechanism of Injury

- Usually result from a direct blow to hand.
- A "boxer's fracture" of the fifth metacarpal neck results from punching an object or person (Figure 9-1).

## Evaluation

- Patient presents complaining of pain or swelling following trauma.
- Assess tenderness, ecchymosis, or swelling at the site of the injury.
- A "loss of knuckle" might be observed with shaft fractures.
- Evaluate for scissoring of digits by asking the patient to flex digits into a fist slowly (Figure 9-2).
- The integrity of the skin can be compromised if the hand punched a tooth; this "fight bite" must be treated with special care (see Chapter 30).
- Assess AP, lateral, and oblique radiographs of the hand for the presence of fracture(s), angulation, rotation, displacement, or intra-articular extension.
- The base of the metacarpal must be evaluated to ensure there is no carpometacarpal dislocation; this is noted when the 4 metacarpals are not aligned in parallel on a lateral radiograph (Figure 9-3).

**Figure 9-1.** Radiographs (AP, lateral, and oblique) of a "boxer's fracture."

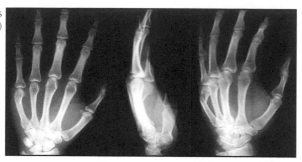

**Figure 9-2.** Malrotation of ring digit due to fourth metacarpal fracture; this "scissoring" will not correct itself, so reduction with or without fixation will be required.

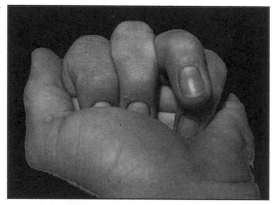

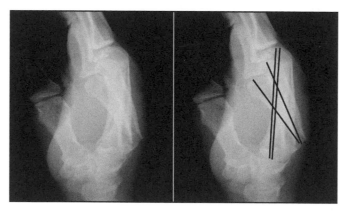

**Figure 9-3.** Metacarpals 2, 3, 4, and 5 should align in parallel on a lateral radiograph. This lateral radiograph demonstrates that two of the metacarpals are not parallel to the other two; note the fractures at the bases of these metacarpals.

## Acute Treatment

- Apply a volar splint with the hand in position of function, or an ulnar gutter splint if the fracture involves the fourth or fifth metacarpal.
- Reduction of metacarpal neck fractures (most likely in the fifth metacarpal, or boxer's fracture) can be accomplished by volar pressure on the metacarpal head.

## Definitive Treatment (Refer to Hand Specialist)

- If the fracture is nondisplaced and considered stable, the injury likely can be treated with immobilization, followed by controlled range of motion.
- If the fracture is displaced or unstable, appropriate treatment might require closed reduction and percutaneous pinning (CRPP), or open reduction and internal fixation (ORIF).

## Potential Problems

- Healing in the "wrong position" (malunion) can cause scissoring or dysfunction of the tendon mechanism.
- Failure to heal (nonunion) is rare but can occur.

## Special Consideration: Bennett Fracture

- The Bennett Fracture is an intra-articular fracture at the base of the thumb metacarpal (Figure 9-4).
- This fracture occurs from an axial force through a semi-flexed metacarpal; the metacarpal shaft is displaced radially and dorsally by the pull of the multiple tendons, while the volar ulnar fragment of the joint surface remains in place.
- A thumb spica splint is applied in the urgent situation.
- If there is displacement, a hand surgeon will perform CRPP or ORIF.
- Immobilization for at least 6 weeks is expected.
- The Rolando variant is a T- or Y-shaped intra-articular fracture at the base of the first metacarpal; these also require CRPP or ORIF.

**Figure 9-4.** Displaced Bennett fracture at base of thumb metacarpal.

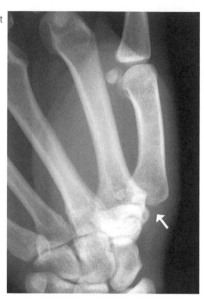

## SUGGESTED READING

Kozin SH, Thoder JJ, Lieberman G. Operative treatment of metacarpal and phalangeal shaft fractures. *J Am Acad Orthop Surg.* 2000;8(2):111-121.

Lee SG, Jupiter JB. Phalangeal and metacarpal fractures of the hand. *Hand Clin.* 2000;16(3):323-332.

Soyer AD. Fractures of the base of the first metacarpal: current treatment options. *J Am Acad Orthop Surg.* 1999;7(6):403-412.

# chapter 10

# SCAPHOID FRACTURES

Scaphoid fractures account for approximately 60% of all carpal bone fractures. They often are misdiagnosed as a simple "wrist sprain." Unfortunately, these missed injuries go on to malunion or nonunion, resulting in persistent wrist pain and wrist arthritis. Therefore, if there is any question at all, it is best to treat as if there is a fracture and refer early.

## Mechanism of Injury

- Most often results from a fall onto an outstretched hand, usually when patient lands with wrist extended and radially deviated.
- Also can occur by blunt axial load (eg, blocking by football lineman).

## Evaluation

- Patient might have tenderness to palpation, swelling in anatom ic snuffbox (Figure 10-1), tenderness volarly at scaphoid distal pole, or report pain with axial compression of the thumb.
- Assess AP, lateral, oblique, and scaphoid (ulnar deviation) radiographic views of the wrist (Figure 10-2).

## Acute Treatment

- Immobilize in well-padded thumb spica splint.
- If no fracture is identified radiographically, but the clinical

**Figure 10-1.** The "anatomic snuffbox" is the area bounded by the extensor pollicis brevis (first dorsal compartment) and extensor pollicis longus (third dorsal compartment); tenderness in this area can be associated with scaphoid fractures.

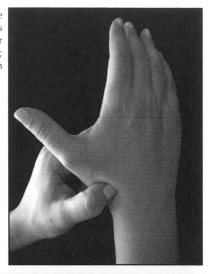

**Figure 10-2.** This 18-year-old right-hand-dominant female pedestrian was struck by a car and fell onto her right hand. Initial radiographs in the emergency room (A and B) did not demonstrate a fracture. A dedicated scaphoid (ulnar deviation) radiograph (C), however, clearly shows the scaphoid wrist fracture.

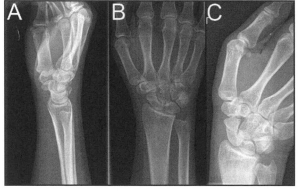

exam is suspicious, treat the patient as if he or she has a fracture, and repeat radiographs in 2 weeks.

## Definitive Treatment (Refer to Hand Specialist)

- Nondisplaced fractures can be treated surgically via percutaneous screw fixation (Figure 10-3) or in a thumb spica cast.
- Displaced fractures (>1 mm) require surgical reduction and fixation.
- Healing usually takes at least 6 to 12 weeks.

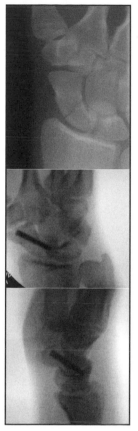

**Figure 10-3.** This scaphoid fracture was treated with percutaneous screw fixation, allowing protected early range of motion activities.

## Potential Problems

- Malunion and nonunion rates are significant, particularly if the injury is missed or not treated; both instances can lead to long-term wrist pain and arthritis.
- Return to work can be delayed weeks to months, depending on the patient's occupational demands.

### Suggested Reading

Haisman JM, Rohde RS, Weiland AJ. Acute fractures of the scaphoid. *J Bone Joint Surg Am.* 2006;88(12):2750-2758.
Plancher KD. Methods of imaging the scaphoid. *Hand Clin.* 2001;17(4):703-721.

# chapter 11

# CARPAL (NON-SCAPHOID) FRACTURES

Non-scaphoid fractures account for about 30% to 40% of carpal bone fractures.

## Triquetral Fracture

### Mechanism of Injury

- Most commonly fractured carpal bone other than the scaphoid
- "Shear" fracture from extreme dorsiflexion of triquetrum against ulnar styloid (usually from a fall onto an outstretched hand)

### Evaluation

- Tenderness in dorsal ulnar hand/carpus
- Radiographs show "chip" fracture dorsal to triquetrum (Figure 11-1).

### Acute Treatment

- Cast or splint immobilization

### Definitive Treatment

- Immobilization for 4 to 6 weeks or symptomatic treatment

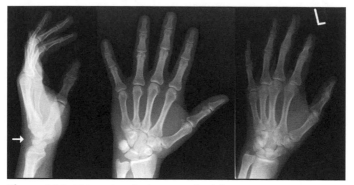

**Figure 11-1.** This patient had sustained a fall onto an outstretched left hand. Three radiographic views of his hand were obtained. The triquetral avulsion fracture is only visible on the lateral view, as indicated by the arrow (left).

## Potential Problems

- Persistent pain

## *Hook of Hamate Fracture*

### Mechanism of Injury

- Racquet or club sports (especially golf and baseball) injury resulting from direct impact on hamate hook in palm

### Evaluation

- Ulnar sided hand/wrist pain, tenderness to palpation at hook of hamate, pain with resisted flexion of ring and small fingers
- Radiographs of hand, including carpal tunnel view (Figure 11-2)
- Computed tomography (CT) scan of hands in "praying position."

### Acute Treatment

- Cast immobilization

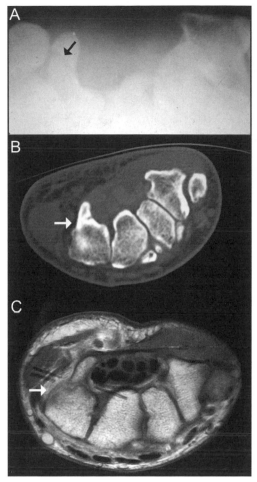

**Figure 11-2.** Radiograph (A), axial CT scan image (B), and axial MRI image (C) of 3 different patients with hamate hook fractures. The carpal tunnel radiograph is the first-line diagnostic study if this fracture is suspected. The CT scan can be performed if the carpal tunnel view does not show a fracture but suspicion is high. MRI generally is not used for this, but this patient underwent MRI for "wrist pain" and was found to have this hamate hook nonunion.

## Definitive Treatment

- Cast immobilization rarely leads to union.
- Excision of the hamate hook is performed for the vast majority of symptomatic fracture nonunions.

## Potential Problems

- Rough edges on the fracture can lead to ring and small finger flexor tendon ruptures.

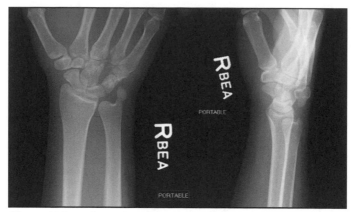

**Figure 11-3.** Radiographs of this wrist demonstrate fracture-dislocations of the hamate and fourth and fifth metacarpal bases.

- Nonunion is common; if symptomatic, the hook can be excised electively.

## Hamate Body Fractures

### Mechanism of Injury

- Axial load on clenched fist, usually accompanies dislocation of the fourth or fifth CMC joints

### Evaluation

- Pain and deformity at fourth and fifth CMC joints and hamate
- Radiographs of hand, lateral view demonstrates dorsal migration of metacarpal bases with hamate (Figure 11-3).

### Acute Treatment

- Splint for comfort and refer as soon as possible; the inherent instability of this injury makes it likely that surgery will be required.

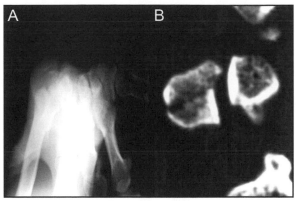

**Figure 11-4.** Radiograph (A) and sagittal CT scan image (B) of a pisiform fracture in a professional baseball player who sustained a direct blow to the palmar ulnar side of his carpus.

## Definitive Treatment

- Closed reduction and percutaneous screw fixation, or ORIF

## Potential Problems

- Nonunion, arthritis (pain)

### Pisiform Fractures

## Mechanism of Injury

- Direct blow to ulnar side of hand

## Evaluation

- Tenderness to palpation of pisiform
- Evaluate for ulnar nerve dysfunction
- Radiographs of hand, including carpal tunnel view (Figure 11-4A) or slightly supinated lateral of the wrist to profile the pisiform

- CT scan can be helpful if radiographs do not show fracture (Figure 11-4B)

## Acute Treatment

- Cast immobilization

## Definitive Treatment

- Usually cast immobilization is sufficient, but a symptomatic nonunion or displaced fracture can be treated by excision.

## Potential Problems

- Ulnar nerve dysfunction, persistent pain

### *Capitate Fractures*

Isolated capitate fractures are extremely rare (1% of carpal bone fractures); these more often are associated with perilunate dislocations.

## Mechanism of Injury

- Direct blow or forced dorsiflexion of wrist

## Evaluation

- Tenderness, swelling of carpal area
- Radiographs of hand

## Acute Treatment

- Splint immobilization

## Definitive Treatment

- Cast immobilization if nondisplaced, ORIF if displaced

## Lunate, Trapezium, and Trapezoid Fractures

These fractures are very rare; as long as a perilunate injury has been excluded, the hand and wrist can be immobilized and the patient referred to a hand specialist within a few days.

### SUGGESTED READING

Papp S. Carpal bone fractures. *Orthop Clin North Am.* 2007;38(2):251-260.

Vigler M, Aviles A, Lee SK. Carpal fractures excluding the scaphoid. *Hand Clin.* 2006;22(4):501-516.

# chapter 12

# PERILUNATE DISLOCATIONS

Perilunate dislocations are high-energy injuries that reportedly are missed 25% of the time. They are associated with disruption of multiple intercarpal ligaments and can involve fractures and median nerve injury.

## Mechanism of Injury

- Usually a result of high energy injuries (eg, motor vehicle accident)
- Can occur following a fall (especially from height)
- Generally caused by hyperextension of the wrist

## Evaluation

- Patient might present with multiple injuries from the traumatic event.
- Complaint of severe pain, possibly swelling
- Diffuse tenderness about the wrist can be difficult to localize
- Wrist and digital range of motion limited
- Evaluate median nerve sensation; acute carpal tunnel syndrome can result from the lunate compressing the median nerve.
- Assess entire upper extremity for concomitant injuries.
- Radiographs: assess AP, lateral, oblique, and scaphoid views
- Lateral radiograph shows that radius, lunate, capitate, and third metacarpal are not aligned; might show "teacup sign" (Figure 12-1).
- Can be accompanied by scaphoid or radial styloid fractures

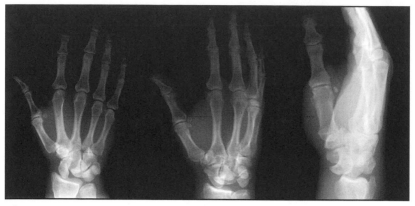

**Figure 12-1.** Following a fall from a 15-foot ladder, this patient was brought to the emergency room with obvious facial injuries but complaining of right hand pain and progressive "numbness" in his median nerve distribution. Radiographs, particularly the lateral view, demonstrate dislocation of the lunate palmarly. Note the "spilled teacup sign" of the lunate on the lateral view. The lunate was compressing the median nerve. This patient was brought to the operating room urgently for carpal tunnel release, open reduction of the dislocation, fixation, and ligamentous repair.

## Acute Treatment

- Initial management involves an attempt at closed reduction, which only should be performed by a trained, comfortable provider. Finger trap traction (10 pounds) is applied for 10 minutes. Dorsiflexion of the wrist, followed by volar flexion while volar pressure is placed on the lunate, can reduce the dislocation. If reduction is attempted, post-reduction radiographs should be performed to confirm successful reduction.
- Apply well-padded plaster volar splint.
- Consult hand surgeon immediately.

## Definitive Treatment (Refer to Hand Specialist)

- Closed reduction is sometimes possible before swelling occurs and requires adequate relaxation, time, and traction.
- Although primary compression of the median nerve occurs at the time of injury, urgent carpal tunnel release is performed if median nerve symptoms are worsening or if closed

reduction is not able to be achieved and urgent open reduction is planned.

• Open reduction and fixation and stabilization of the injury follows.

## Potential Problems

• This is a commonly missed diagnosis and delayed treatment impairs outcome; pain, arthritis, and median neuropathy can develop.

• Pressure on the median nerve can cause permanent neuropathy.

• Even after treatment by the most experienced surgeon, patients can lose wrist range of motion and grip strength.

*SUGGESTED READING*

Grabow RJ, Catalano L III. Carpal dislocations. *Hand Clin.* 2006;22(4):485-500.

Kozin SH. Perilunate injuries: diagnosis and treatment. *J Am Acad Orthop Surg.* 1998;6:114-120.

Sauder DJ, Athwal GS, Roth JH. Perilunate injuries. *Orthop Clin North Am.* 2007;38(2):279-288.

# chapter 13

# DISTAL RADIUS FRACTURES

The distal radius is one of the most commonly fractured bones. Treatment of this "wrist fracture" depends upon patient factors, fracture/bone characteristics, and surgeon preferences.

## Mechanism of Injury

- The most common low-energy mechanism is a fall onto an outstretched hand.
- High-energy mechanisms (eg, motor vehicle accidents, fall from height) tend to result in more comminution, displacement, and associated injuries and typically are less stable because of destruction of the surrounding soft tissue envelope.

## Evaluation

- Inspect for skin lacerations, deformity, swelling, tenderness.
- Remove any rings from the fingers.
- Always keep in mind compartment syndrome as a possible complication.
- Evaluate 2-point discrimination—sensation (especially median nerve area), and motor function of each tendon (these can be associated with tendon ruptures).
- Radiographs should include an AP, lateral, and oblique of the wrist. Look for radial inclination, radial height, and volar tilt (use the 22/11/11 rule) and associated injuries as they will determine management (Figure 13-1).

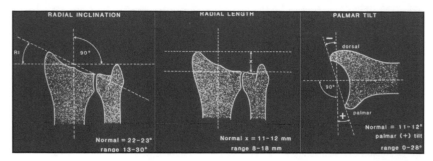

**Figure 13-1.** Radiographs can be used to measure radial inclination, length (or "height"), and palmar tilt of the distal radius. Fractures can cause these to differ from what are considered to be "anatomic." Considerable differences have been shown to lead to poor outcomes in the future, and reduction with or without fixation might be considered.

## Acute Treatment

- If there is an open wound at the fracture site, administer antibiotics and tetanus (if indicated), irrigate the wound, immobilize, and refer urgently to a hand surgeon.
- Nondisplaced fractures can be immobilized in a volar plaster splint and referred (usually within a week). If a cast is applied, bivalve the cast with a cast saw to allow for swelling.
- If there is a radial styloid component, add a thumb spica component to the splint.
- Displaced fractures should be treated by closed reduction and splinting if you are trained and comfortable; if not, refer early (within 1 or 2 days) for closed reduction and further management. A neurological deficit is an indication for urgent referral.
- The patient should be instructed to elevate the hand and wrist above the heart at all times to decrease swelling, and to continue to make a fist and extend digits to prevent stiffness.

## Definitive Treatment (Refer to Hand Specialist)

- Nondisplaced or adequately reduced fractures can be treated with immobilization and careful, frequent follow-up assessments to ensure maintained alignment. High-energy injuries tend to lose reduction and require internal fixation.

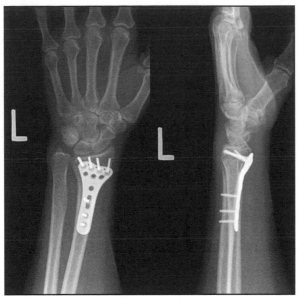

**Figure 13-2.** Radiographs of a distal radius fracture treated with open reduction and internal fixation using a volar plate.

- Difficult to reduce fractures sometimes are treated by a combination of closed or open reduction and immobilization, pinning, internal or external fixation (Figures 13-2 and 13-3) depending on patient and injury variables and surgeon comfort and preference.
- Hand therapy is instituted early to promote digital range of motion.

## Potential Problems

- Nondisplaced fractures are associated with extensor pollicis longus (EPL) ruptures because of bleeding in the nondisrupted tendon sheath, which causes loss of blood supply to the tendon (8.5% incidence).
- Digital and wrist stiffness and distal ulnar pain are common and can be improved by hand therapy.
- Fracture malunion (healing incorrectly) can impede motion and function and cause pain.
- Distal radius fractures can be associated with chronic pain syndromes; patients need to be monitored carefully and treated early if signs of this develop.

**Figure 13-3.** External fixators can be used for maintaining reduction of fractures with dorsal and volar comminution.

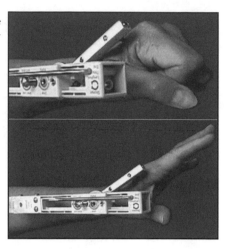

### SUGGESTED READING

Ilyas AM, Jupiter JB. Distal radius fractures—classification of treatment and indications for surgery. *Orthop Clin North Am.* 2007;38(2):167-173.

Turner RG, Faber KJ, Athwal GS. Complications of distal radius fractures. *Orthop Clin North Am.* 2007;38(2):217-228.

Wulf CA, Ackerman DB, Rizzo M. Contemporary evaluation and treatment of distal radius fractures. *Hand Clin.* 2007;23(2):209-226.

# chapter 14

# COMPARTMENT SYNDROME

Compartment syndrome is one of the most emergent orthopedic conditions. As soon as the diagnosis is made, preparations for surgical intervention should begin. Sixty-eight percent of patients undergoing fasciotomy within 12 hours of symptom onset had functional extremities compared to only 8% treated after 12 hours, so it is important not to delay.

## Mechanism of Injury

- Most often a result of edema following a crush by or between heavy objects, also after burns
- Rarely can result from excessive fluid from "outside" sources (intravenous [IV] infiltrate)
- Essentially, anything that increases the pressure inside the small compartments of the hand or decreases the volume available for swelling can cause compartment syndrome.

## Evaluation

- The main sign of compartment syndrome is "pain out of proportion to injury."
- Paresthesias, tense swelling, weakness, and pain with passive motion of the fingers can be present.
- It is rare to find a pulseless limb except in the case of vascular injury or occlusion.
- In obtunded patients or in the setting of equivocal examination, compartment pressures can be measured using a com-

mercial hand-held transducer or an arterial pressure monitoring line attached to a needle inserted into each compartment (usually 25 to 30 mmHg is an indication for surgery in these patients).

- Hand compartment syndromes can present as aching following injury or even repetitive strenuous activity; signs include swelling and loss of digital motion with MCP joints extended and PIP joints flexed.

## Acute Treatment

- Compartment syndrome is a surgical emergency.
- Contact a hand surgeon (or orthopedic trauma surgeon, depending on the policy of your hospital) immediately.
- Remove any constrictive dressings that might be constraining the swelling.
- Discontinue any fluids flowing into that extremity.
- Keep patient NPO (nothing by mouth), and begin preoperative preparation.

## Definitive Treatment (Refer to Hand Specialist)

- The surgeon likely will take the patient to the operating room for emergent fasciotomies (incisions that allow the pressure to dissipate from the tissues).
- The patient will be monitored for associate problems and might require further medical or surgical intervention.

## Potential Problems

- Delayed treatment can lead to tissue necrosis, resulting in irreversible nerve or muscle injury and associated deficits.
- Rhabdomyolosis, renal failure, and other systemic problems can result if the patient is not adequately treated and monitored.

## SUGGESTED READING

Gellman H, Buch K. Acute compartment syndrome of the arm. *Hand Clin.* 1998;14(3):385-389.

Oullette EA. Compartment syndromes in obtunded patients. *Hand Clin.* 1998;14(3):431-450.

# Section III

## Tendon Injuries

# chapter 15

# EXTENSOR TENDON LACERATIONS

Extensor tendon lacerations can be caused by injuries to the dorsum of the hand and wrist. The extensor tendons are divided into 6 dorsal compartments at the level of the wrist. Visualizing the tendons and their routes from each compartment will help you examine and predict lacerations. Extensor tendon injuries are classified according to the level at which the tendon is affected (Figure 15-1).

## Mechanism of Injury

- These can result from lacerations by a knife, glass, saw, or other sharp object.
- Beware of "fist through window" injuries; these often result in much more damage than the superficial lacerations might suggest.

## Evaluation

- Document a thorough examination including wound characteristics (contamination, viability of edges), motion deficits (indicating tendon injury), and, if the tendon is visible through the laceration, the extent of laceration if partial. Do not be fooled by other structures into thinking that a tendon is "intact." When in doubt, assume there is a laceration requiring repair.
- Assess radiographs to look for a foreign body or associated fracture.

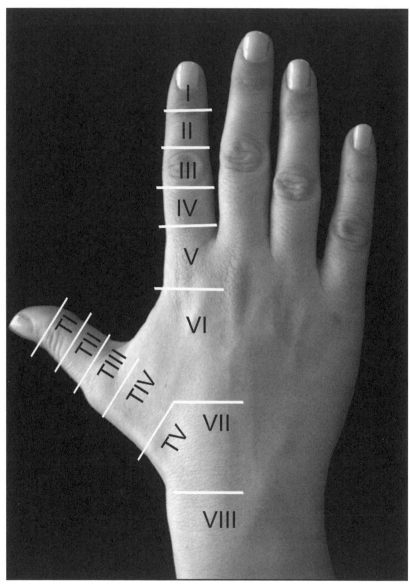

**Figure 15-1.** Extensor tendon lacerations can be classified according to zones: I) DIP joint (TI, IP joint in thumb); II) middle phalanx (TII, proximal phalanx in thumb); III) PIP joint (TIII, MCP joint in thumb); IV) proximal phalanx (TIV, thumb metacarpal); V) MCP joint (TV, CMC joint in thumb); VI) metacarpal; VII) extensor retinaculum; VIII) distal forearm; and IX) forearm (not shown).

## Acute Treatment

- Administer tetanus and antibiotics if indicated.
- Irrigate wound, approximate skin edges with 5-0 nylon suture.
- Splint with wrist in about 20° to 30° of extension, and digits fully extended (including metacarpophalangeal joints), to prevent retraction of proximal tendon stump.
- Refer as soon as possible for repair. If a hand surgeon is immediately available, repair sometimes can be performed under local anesthesia in an outpatient or emergency room setting.

## Definitive Treatment (Refer to Hand Specialist)

- Tendon laceration and other accompanying injuries will be repaired; if the tendon has lost length due to maceration or burn, the patient might require a tendon graft or transfer.
- Patient undergoes splinting and a therapy regimen depending on the location of the laceration.
- In general, extensor tendon repairs are easier to rehabilitate than flexor tendon repairs.

## Potential Problems

- Infection and rupture of the repair are possible.
- Patients can have loss of range of motion—flexion or extension—secondary to scarring.

### SUGGESTED READING

Patel J, Couli R, Harris PA, Percival NJ. Hand lacerations. An audit of clinical examination. *J Hand Surg [Br]*. 1998;23(4):482-484.

Tuncali D, Yavuz N, Terzioglu A, Aslan G. The rate of upper-extremity deep-structure injuries through small penetrating lacerations. *Ann Plast Surg*. 2005;55(2):146-148.

# chapter 16

# *FLEXOR TENDON LACERATIONS*

Flexor tendon lacerations can be some of the worst hand injuries to treat and from which to recover. They are classified as occurring within 1 of 5 zones (Figure 16-1), according to where the tendon injury occurs. Zone 2, where the flexor digitorum superficialis (FDS) and flexor digitorum profundus (FDP) tendons are within the tendon sheath, is called "no man's land" because repairs in the midst of the intricate pulley system here tend to do relatively poorly because of scarring. As a result, patients need to know that although tendon lacerations in the digits generally can be repaired, function following repair will not be completely normal.

## Mechanism of Injury

- Knife, glass, or saw—any sharp object—across the flexor surface can result in tendon laceration.
- Even an apparently minor puncture wound can result in a flexor tendon laceration when the injury occurs with the fingers in flexion.

## Evaluation

- Obtain the details of the injury; in particular, knowing how the digits were positioned (flexion, extension) when injured can help one determine the level of the tendon lacerations (the tendon laceration often is not just under the skin laceration).
- The affected finger rests in an extended posture at one or more joints, depending on which tendon or tendons are lacerated (Figure 16-2).

**Figure 16-1.** Flexor tendon lacerations can be classified by 5 zones: I) distal to the insertion of the FDS tendons; II) FDS insertion to lumbrical origin, included in sheath, also known as "no man's land;" III) origin of lumbricals from FDP tendons; IV) within the carpal tunnel; and V) proximal to the carpal tunnel.

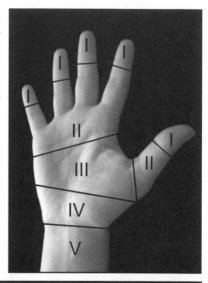

**Figure 16-2.** This 15-year-old right-handed male accidentally cut his left index finger while opening a package with a knife. The relatively extended resting posture (top) indicates laceration of the FDP tendon. He also sustained a laceration of the radial digital nerve. Following repair of the tendon, the digit rests in a more appropriate position (bottom).

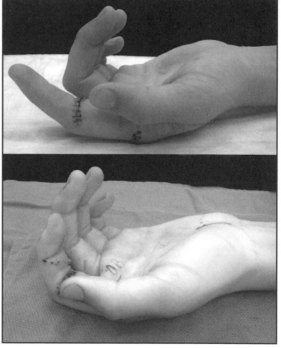

- Test FDS by holding two adjacent fingers extended and asking the patient to flex the PIP joint of the digit being examined.
- Test FDP by asking the patient to flex the digit at the DIP joint.
- Test FPL by asking the patient to flex the thumb at the interphalangeal (IP) joint.
- Document the neurovascular examination because lacerations of the digital nerves and vessels are commonly seen with flexor tendon lacerations.
- Assess radiographs for foreign body or concomitant fracture.

## Acute Treatment

- Administer antibiotics and tetanus if indicated.
- Irrigate the wound and close the skin using 5-0 nylon suture.
- Do not use electrocautery or suture ligation to stop digital vessels from bleeding; this can damage the vessel and make it difficult or impossible to repair if needed. Also, the vessel is in close proximity to the digital nerve, and attempts to ligate or cauterize the vessel can damage the adjacent nerve.
- Splint the wrist and digits with a dorsal blocking splint to prevent extension with retraction of proximal tendon stump.
- Instruct the patient not to continue to try to flex the digit as this can cause tendon retraction proximally and complicate repair.
- Refer as soon as possible to a hand surgeon for evaluation and repair.

## Definitive Treatment (Refer to Hand Specialist)

- Most hand surgeons will repair flexor tendon lacerations within a few days of injury.
- Digital nerve repair, if necessary, can be completed at the same time.
- Patients generally will require weeks to months of splinting and supervised hand therapy.
- Outcomes following tendon repair vary greatly, and are particularly dependent upon the location of the laceration (again, zone 2 injuries are the worst).

## Potential Problems

- The most common complication is scarring (adhesion formation), which causes stiffness, decreased range of motion, and pain.
- Rupture of the tendon repair is possible.
- Joint contracture and pulley injury, resulting in "bowstringing" of the tendons, can occur.
- Other digit deformities and motion hindrances can be observed following this injury.
- Delayed diagnosis or treatment can complicate primary repair and necessitate staged tendon reconstruction.

*SUGGESTED READING*

Beredjiklian PK. Biologic aspects of flexor tendon laceration and repair. *J Bone Joint Surg Am.* 2003;85-A(3):539-550.

Lilly SI, Messer TM. Complications after treatment of flexor tendon injuries. *J Am Acad Orthop Surg.* 2006;14(7):387-396.

# chapter 17

# EXTENSOR TENDON AVULSIONS (MALLET FINGER)

The term "mallet finger" was coined to describe the appearance of this common sports-related finger injury in the 1800s. Doyle classified mallet fingers into 4 categories: closed (I), open laceration (II), open abrasion (III), and mallet fracture (IV). As one would expect, the presentation of mallet finger is very similar to that of "mallet fracture," or Type IV mallet finger. A "tendon-only" mallet finger involves avulsion of the extensor tendon only, without part of the distal phalanx.

## Mechanism of Injury

- Forced extension of the distal phalanx against resistance causes the extensor tendon to avulse from the distal phalanx without bone fragment.
- This injury commonly occurs in sports when a ball hits the dorsum of the fingertip (sometimes called "baseball finger").
- Tendon avulsion also happens with activities of daily living, such as tucking a shirt into pants, or tucking sheets under a bed mattress.
- Open injuries to the distal dorsal digit can result in extensor tendon laceration or maceration.

## Evaluation

- Like in mallet fractures, patients usually present with complaints of an inability to straighten a finger (see Figure 4-1).

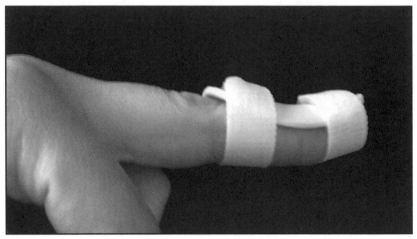

**Figure 17-1.** Mallet finger is treated by holding the DIP joint in hyperextension for an extended period, allowing the extensor tendon to heal back to the distal phalanx.

- The digit rests with the DIP joint in flexion, and the patient is unable to extend actively at the DIP joint.
- Open injuries affecting the dorsum of the DIP joint should raise suspicion for extensor tendon injury, confirmed by inability to extend the DIP joint actively.
- Unlike mallet fracture, radiographs reveal only the flexed posture of the digit without avulsion fracture fragment.

## Acute Treatment

- Splint the DIP joint in hyperextension (Figure 17-1). If a Stax splint is available, that can be used. Otherwise, an aluminum-foam splint can be molded to create hyperextension at the DIP joint.
- Inform the patient that this needs to stay on at all times until he or she sees the hand specialist. Removing the splint and letting the joint bend, even briefly, tears off the tendon and resets the clock to zero.
- Open injuries require irrigation and repair; abrasion injuries might require staged reconstruction if there is considerable soft tissue loss or exposed bone.

## Definitive Treatment (Refer to Hand Specialist)

- Acute Type I mallet fingers can be treated closed in a DIP hyperextension splint for 6 to 8 weeks. Well-fitting splints are fabricated by hand therapists, who also instruct the patient regarding skin care and splinting regimen.
- Patients who cannot perform their occupation with a splint (eg, surgeons, musicians) might be candidates for temporary placement of a percutaneous "pin" across the joint to serve as an "internal splint."
- Patients are checked periodically clinically to ensure the splint is fitting appropriately and that there is no skin breakdown.
- Acute Type II and III mallet fingers are rare but usually are treated surgically with one or more procedures. Pinning of the DIP joint in extension might be performed simultaneously to facilitate wound care.

## Potential Problems

- DIP hyperextension splints are cumbersome, and patients often remove them; removal and allowance of the joint to flex resets the 6- to 8-week clock back to time zero.
- Skin breakdown can occur with splinting.
- An extensor lag of 5° to 10° at the DIP joint is not uncommon following treatment.
- Many hand surgeons consider presentation 4 weeks following injury "chronic," although patients usually can be treated nonoperatively for several weeks longer than that. However, some of these might not heal without surgery. If left too long, the patient can develop compensatory deformity of the digit because the tendon balance is affected (swan neck deformity).

### SUGGESTED READING

Bendre AA, Hartigan BJ, Kalainov DM. Mallet finger. *J Am Acad Orthop Surg.* 2005;13(5):336-344.

Tuttle HG, Olvey SP, Stern PJ. Tendon avulsion injuries of the distal phalanx. *Clin Orthop Rel Res.* 2006;445:157-168.

# chapter 18

# FLEXOR TENDON AVULSIONS (JERSEY FINGER)

"Jersey finger" is the common name for avulsion of the FDP tendon from the distal phalanx, resulting in inability to flex the DIP joint. This is commonly missed because "X-rays are negative" and misdiagnosed as a sprain. Depending on the extent of retraction of the tendon, the tendon sometimes loses its blood supply and becomes necrotic as time passes. If these injuries are not recognized and treated surgically within 7 to 10 days, primary repair might not be possible.

## Mechanism of Injury

- Forced extension of a flexed digit results in rupture of the FDP tendon from the volar aspect of the distal phalanx.
- The name "jersey finger" was coined because this injury can occur when a player's digit gets caught in another player's jersey. It also is known to happen when a finger gets caught in a basketball net and is flexed against the resistance of the net.
- Seventy-five percent of these injuries occur in the ring finger; multiple reasons for this have been proposed in the literature. With fingers flexed, the ring finger is the longest digit and absorbs the maximum force.

## Evaluation

- DIP joint of the affected digit rests in extension (Figure 18-1).
- Patient is unable to flex DIP joint of digit actively.

85

**Figure 18-1.** Ring finger FDP avulsion in a 14-year-old male who caught the digit on a basketball net. Note the extended posture of the ring finger DIP joint relative to that of the other digits.

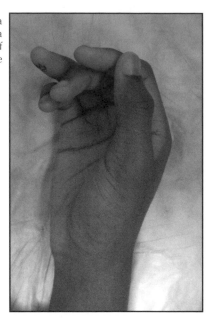

- Palpating fullness at the PIP joint or MCP joint can help identify to what extent the tendon has retracted; the patient also might have tenderness at the level of retraction.
- Radiographs (especially lateral) can identify an avulsed fracture fragment and help localize the extent of retraction. Subluxation of the distal phalanx dorsally also should be assessed.

## Acute Treatment

- Immobilize hand and wrist with wrist in neutral or slightly flexed, MCP joints flexed, digits flexed in comfort to prevent further retraction of tendons.
- Recommend ice, rest, elevation, and early referral to a hand surgeon (preferably within 1 or 2 days).
- It is crucial to explain the importance of early follow-up and treatment to the patient.

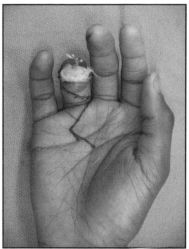

**Figure 18-2.** The FDP tendon was reinserted through the pulley system and attached to the distal phalanx using sutures that pull through the nail plate and are tied over a button. The hand is splinted with a splint that does not allow the digit to extend fully (potentially jeopardizing the repair) and the patient begins supervised motion with a hand therapist. The button is removed at around 6 weeks postoperatively.

## Definitive Treatment (Refer to Hand Specialist)

- Surgical repair either with a suture anchor, a screw (in case of large fracture fragment), or suture over a button is performed as soon as possible, usually within 7 to 10 days (Figure 18-2).
- Delayed treatment can necessitate staged reconstruction or salvage procedures (multiple surgeries, prolonged recovery, worse outcome).

## Potential Problems

- Patients should expect a decreased range of motion at the DIP joint following repair.
- The patient might need a more extensive procedure if treated late (possibly even by 10 days).
- Arthritis of the DIP joint can develop if the avulsion fracture fragment is relatively large.

### SUGGESTED READING

Stamos BD, Leddy JP. Closed flexor tendon disruption in athletes. *Hand Clin.* 2000;16(3):359-365.

Tuttle HG, Olvey SP, Stern PJ. Tendon avulsion injuries of the distal phalanx. *Clin Orthop Rel Res.* 2006;445:157-168.

# Section IV

## Nerve Injuries

# chapter 19

# DIGITAL NERVE INJURIES

Usually resulting from lacerations, digital nerve injuries commonly are missed. Even a superficial laceration can result in transection of a digital nerve. Prompt identification of this injury, and referral for possible surgical repair, can lead to an improved outcome.

## Mechanism of Injury

- These usually result from lacerations, particularly those along the sides of the palmar digit or the palmar aspect of the MCP joint.
- In the finger, the nerve is volar (palmar) to the blood vessels. If the finger is cut, it hurts before it bleeds.
- Blunt injury can cause neuropraxia, a kind of stretch injury.

## Evaluation

- Assess extent and location of laceration.
- Each digit has a nerve on the radial and ulnar sides and there can be overlap of sensory areas; evaluate 2-point discrimination on each side of the fingertip pulp and document paresthesias and sensory loss.
- Associated injuries include vascular injury (check capillary refill or digital Doppler), tendon lacerations, and fractures.

**Figure 19-1.** This patient sustained an open fracture from a crush injury which resulted in neuropraxia; digital nerve exploration revealed continuity of the nerve. The patient ultimately recovered full sensation with normal 2-point discrimination in the area supplied by this nerve.

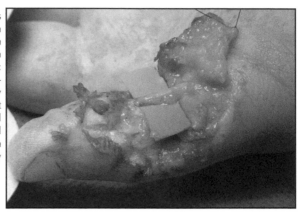

## Acute Treatment

- Administer tetanus and antibiotics if indicated.
- Irrigate and close skin with 5-0 nylon suture (or absorbable suture in children), apply sterile dressings and a well-padded plaster splint (particularly according to other injuries like tendon laceration or fracture).
- Patients might have complete transection of the nerve (requiring repair) or a "stretch" (neuropraxia), which recovers with observation (Figure 19-1).
- Refer to hand surgeon within the next few days.

## Definitive Treatment (Refer to Hand Specialist)

- Digital nerve lacerations are repaired using magnification as soon as possible but not necessarily urgently.
- Recovery of sensation depends greatly on the patient's age; younger patients (<20) tend to recover better than older patients. Nerve recovery generally begins after the first month and is expected to occur at a rate of approximately 1 mm per day.

## Potential Problems

- Neuroma, or painful nerve ending, can occur.
- Failure to recover sensation becomes more likely with the increased age of the patient.

### SUGGESTED READING

Goldie BS, Coates CJ, Birch R. The long term result of digital nerve repair in no-man's land. *J Hand Surg [Br]*. 1992;17B:75-77.

Siddiqui A, Benjamin CI, Schubert W. Incidence of neurapraxia in digital nerve injuries. *J Reconstr Microsurg*. 2000;16(2):95-98.

chapter 20

# MEDIAN NERVE INJURIES

The median nerve supplies motor innervation to most of the flexor muscles in the forearm and to several of the intrinsic muscles in the hand (the radial two lumbricals, opponens pollicis, abductor pollicis, and half of flexor pollicis brevis). It also supplies sensory innervation to the radial aspect of the palm (via its palmar cutaneous branch) and the thumb, index, long, and radial half of the ring fingers (see Appendix J). The most common median nerve "injury" you will see is carpal tunnel syndrome, which can occur acutely if there has been trauma to the hand and/or wrist. Early recognition and treatment results in improved outcomes.

## Mechanism of Injury

- Hand and wrist fractures or dislocations can cause neuropraxia from tethering or compression.
- Crush injuries with or without fracture or dislocation can result in compartment syndrome or acute swelling in the carpal canal.
- Laceration at the wrist crease—especially transverse (eg, suicide attempt)—often results in median nerve injury.

## Evaluation

- Ask about pain or paresthesias (numbness/tingling) in the median nerve distribution (thumb, index, long, radial aspect of ring).
- Look for lacerations across the midline of the wrist (Figure 20-1) or deformity of the wrist.

95

**Figure 20-1.** This 41-year-old left-hand-dominant man lacerated his right wrist in a suicide attempt. His laceration was closed and he was admitted to a psychiatric unit. Ten days later, he complained of numbness in the thumb, index, and long fingers and a hand surgery evaluation was requested. Intraoperative evaluation revealed complete lacerations of his median nerve and two FDS tendons.

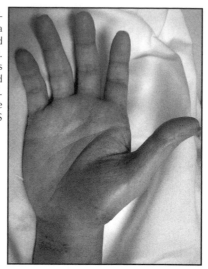

- Severe swelling following a crush injury could be indicative of compartment syndrome (see Chapter 14).
- Check sensation (2-point discrimination) of digits in median nerve distribution.
- If possible, check strength of abduction of thumb, realizing that this might be difficult for a patient in pain.
- Radiographs demonstrating perilunate dislocation (see Chapter 12) or other fracture-dislocations (Figure 20-2) should raise suspicion of median nerve "tenting," compression, or contusion.

## Acute Treatment

- If symptoms are associated with severe bony injury, reduction of the fracture or dislocation should be performed as soon as possible to minimize tethering/compression.
- Start preparing in case urgent surgery is needed (keep NPO, preoperative evaluation).

## Definitive Treatment (Refer to Hand Specialist)

- Acute median nerve injury—whether blunt or sharp—should

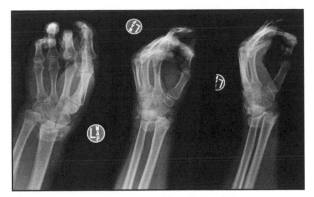

**Figure 20-2.** This 86-year-old right-hand-dominant man and former Green Beret fell from a ladder and sustained this closed injury to his left wrist. He complained primarily of "tingling" in the median nerve distribution. Radiographs show these displaced fractures of the distal radius and ulna; the median nerve likely was tented over the volar "spike" of the diaphyseal ("shaft") fragment. Closed reduction and splinting in the emergency room led to resolution of the symptoms; the patient was taken to the operating room electively for fixation of the fractures days later, at which time he had no persistent median nerve symptoms and thus did not require carpal tunnel release.

be evaluated by a hand surgeon urgently for consideration of surgical intervention.

• Urgent carpal tunnel release and other operative interventions are performed for worsening median nerve symptoms, presence of compressive structure (usually bone) in the carpal canal, or compartment syndrome. If reduction of a fracture or dislocation results in progressive resolution of symptoms, surgery likely can be scheduled "electively" within the next several days.

## Potential Problems

• Functional recovery varies depending on extent and timing of injury and subsequent management.
• Decreased sensation, motor deficits (especially in functioning of the thumb), and chronic pain all are possible.

## SUGGESTED READING

Mack GR, McPherson SA, Lutz RB. Acute median neuropathy after wrist trauma. The role of emergent carpal tunnel release. *Clin Orthop Relat Res.* 1994;(300):141-146.

Szabo RM. Acute carpal tunnel syndrome. *Hand Clin.* 1998;14(3):419-429.

# chapter 21

# ULNAR NERVE INJURIES

The ulnar nerve supplies motor innervation to the ulnar flexors in the forearm and all except the median-innervated muscles in the hand. In addition, it supplies sensory innervation to the small finger and the ulnar half of the ring finger (see Appendix J). The ulnar nerve is particularly vulnerable to superficial lacerations on the ulnar side of the wrist and to penetrating injuries near the hamate hook, where the motor branch of the ulnar nerve comes off of the main nerve.

## Mechanism of Injury

- Penetrating or crush injuries near the hamate hook can damage motor or sensory branches or both.
- The ulnar nerve can be injured by any laceration on the ulnar side of the wrist (Figure 21-1), especially from striking the hand through a sheet of glass. Even small lacerations can involve significant nerve injury.
- Blast injury from a gunshot wound (refer to Chapter 34) usually results in neuropraxia, rather than laceration.

## Evaluation

- Ask about pain or paresthesias (numbness/tingling) in the ulnar-innervated digits.
- Look for lacerations at the ulnar aspect of the wrist or penetrating injuries near hook of hamate, around which the ulnar motor branch lies (Figure 21-1).

**Figure 21-1.** This innocuous-appearing laceration occurred when a 16-year-old right-hand-dominant male punched his right hand through a glass window. However, the entire ulnar nerve was lacerated, as were the extensor carpi ulnaris and the flexor tendons to the small finger (as evidenced by its extended posture).

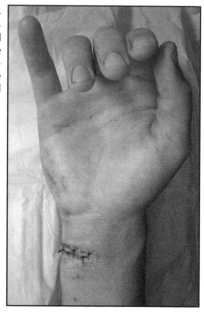

- Check sensation (2-point discrimination ) of digits in ulnar nerve distribution (particularly small finger).

- Examine for ulnar motor function: intrinsics (cross your fingers); evaluate for first dorsal interosseous key pinch ("Froment's sign" is when they cannot key pinch, but use the median innervated flexor pollicis longus [FPL] to bend the IP joint of the thumb instead), clawing (lack of lumbrical function on ring finger and small MCP joints will not allow flexion of the MCP joints). (Figure 21-2)

- Evaluate perfusion of the hand including each individual digit; the ulnar artery or palmar arch might be lacerated as well.

- Radiographs demonstrating hamate injury should raise suspicion for ulnar nerve injury.

- Preserved sensation alone does not guarantee an intact ulnar nerve.

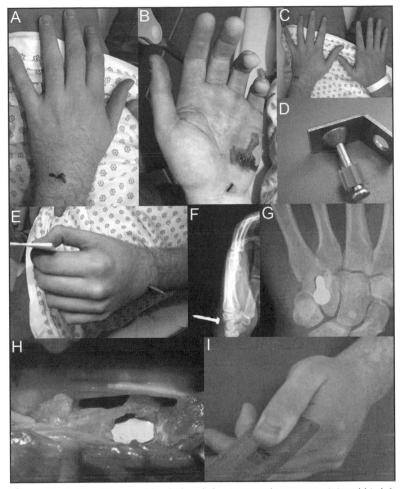

**Figure 21-2.** This 28-year-old right-hand-dominant male carpenter injured his left hand while using a nail gun. He presented with the nail protruding from the dorsum of his hand (A), having entered through the palm (B). When asked to extend his digits, clawing was noted at the ulnar side of the left hand (C). The nail configuration is shown in (D). Further evaluation demonstrated Froment's sign (E), which is when the ulnar-innervated first dorsal interosseous muscle is not functioning, and in order to "pinch" an object between thumb and forefinger, the patient must use the median-innervated FPL muscle. Lateral (F) and AP (G) radiographs show that the nail, and its surrounding orange plastic, traversed through the hamate. Exploration intraoperatively revealed transection of the motor branch of the ulnar nerve, which was repaired (H). Six-month follow-up demonstrated fully functioning ulnar-innervated intrinsic muscles of the hand, as shown by the patient's negative Froment's sign (I).

## Acute Treatment

- Administer tetanus and antibiotics if indicated.
- Irrigate wound if penetration or laceration occurred, particularly if the wound is grossly contaminated.
- Prepare patient for possible surgical intervention (keep NPO, obtain preoperative labs and studies).
- Referral to hand specialist immediately for evaluation and management.

## Definitive Treatment (Refer to Hand Specialist)

- Acute ulnar nerve injury should be evaluated by a hand surgeon urgently for consideration of surgical intervention.
- If vascular injury is present and demonstrates compromised blood flow to a digit or the hand, emergent evaluation by a hand surgeon is necessary.
- The ulnar nerve (or branches) can be repaired. Concomitant injuries can be addressed at the same time. The hand is splinted to immobilize the repair.

## Potential Problems

- Functional recovery varies depending on extent and timing of injury and subsequent management.
- Decreased sensation, motor deficits, and chronic pain all are possible.

*SUGGESTED READING*

Pfaeffle HJ, Waitayawinyu T, Trumble TE. Ulnar nerve laceration and repair. *Hand Clin.* 2007;23(3):291-299.

Waugh RP, Pellegrini VD Jr. Ulnar tunnel syndrome. *Hand Clin.* 2007;23(3):301-310.

# chapter 22

# RADIAL NERVE INJURIES

The radial nerve supplies motor function to most extensor muscles in the upper extremity, including the triceps, brachioradialis, extensor carpi radialis brevis (ECRB), extensor carpi radialis longus (ECRL), extensor pollicis longus (EPL), extensor pollicis brevis (EPB), extensor digitorum communis (EDC), extensor indicis proprius (EIP), extensor digiti quinti (EDQ), and extensor carpi ulnaris (ECU). It branches at the radial neck into the posterior interosseous nerve, which supplies many of the above-listed muscles, and the superficial branch of the radial nerve, which supplies sensory innervation to a large part of the dorsum of the hand (see Appendix J).

## Mechanism of Injury

- Most often, the injury is a neuropraxia accompanying a distal third humerus fracture (85% recover in 3 months).
- Posterior interosseous nerve (PIN) palsy can occur with fractures or dislocations of the radial head.
- Penetrating injuries such as gunshot wounds (refer to Chapter 34) and open fractures may result in transection or neuropraxia.
- Laceration or contusion of the superficial branch of the radial nerve can be found with injury to the dorsum of wrist (Figure 22-1).

## Evaluation

- Assess the site of the traumatic injury; suspect radial nerve injury if trauma occurred at distal humerus, radial head, or radial aspect of the wrist.

**Figure 22-1.** Laceration of the superficial branch of the radial nerve can occur with a penetrating injury (including iatrogenic) to the dorsoradial forearm. This nerve laceration had been missed and was grafted during this procedure.

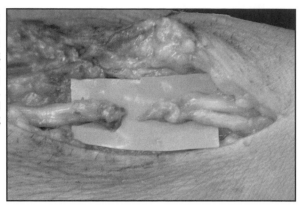

- Evaluate for sensory deficit on dorsum of hand.
- Weakness of wrist extension, digit extension (particularly EPL), "wrist drop," or inability to extend the wrist, might be observed if motor branches are injured.
- Radiographs of the injured site should be assessed.

## Acute Treatment

- Administer tetanus and antibiotics if indicated.
- If there is an open wound, irrigate to remove contamination and prevent infection.
- Immobilize fractures to keep patient comfortable.
- Consult appropriate upper extremity specialist urgently for open injuries or those associated with fracture.

## Definitive Treatment (Refer to Hand Specialist)

- Open fractures usually will be treated urgently with irrigation and debridement, fracture fixation, and possibly exploration of the radial nerve (depending on the nature of the injury).
- Lacerations of the nerve will need to be repaired, grafted, or bridged with a nerve conduit. If the mechanism is high-energy, the surgeon might wait for the extent of nerve injury to declare itself, as often the zone of injury is much larger than it appears initially.

- Contusions of the nerve are observed and recovery potential is high with use of proper splinting and therapy techniques.

## Potential Problems

- Functional recovery depends upon type of injury, associated injuries (fracture, soft tissue deficit, etc), and appropriate management.
- Deficits (wrist drop, lack of finger extension) might occur and would be an indication for possible tendon transfers (4 to 6 months after injury).
- Semi-acute pain (eg, neuroma) or chronic pain syndromes can develop.

*SUGGESTED READING*

Robson AJ, See MS, Ellis H. Applied anatomy of the superficial branch of the radial nerve. *Clin Anat.* 2008;21(1):38-45.

# Section V

## Hand and Wrist Infections

# chapter 23

# *FELON/PULP SPACE INFECTIONS*

A felon is a pulp-space infection of the fingertip. There are many septal compartments in the pulp of the digit; infection results in accumulation of purulence, which increases swelling and pain in the fingertip. Most of these are caused by *Staphylococcus aureus*; unfortunately, methicillin resistant *S. aureus* is becoming more common.

## Mechanism of Injury

- Patient may or may not recall a prior laceration or puncture wound to the fingertip.
- An abscess develops in the pulp space of the digit (Figure 23-1) and pus collects between septa in the pulp.

## Evaluation

- Patient presents complaining of increasing tenderness, swelling, and erythema of fingertip, all of which usually are revealed on examination.
- Identify any puncture wounds on the pulp of the affected digit.
- Radiographs can be used to identify foreign body or fracture (patients with diabetic neuropathy can present with swollen fingertips that appear infected, but actually are fractured, and vice versa).

**Figure 23-1.** Felon infection with erythema and subcutaneous abscess; a mid-lateral incision allows insertion of a hemostat to evacuate septal compartments. (Photo courtesy of Dr. Jeffrey C. King.) *For a full-color version, see page CA-II of the Color Atlas.*

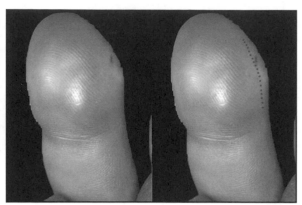

## Acute Treatment

- Warm soaks, elevation, and antibiotics sometimes can lead to resolution of very early symptoms.
- If there is an abscess, incision and debridement is necessary to drain the purulence and allow resolution of the infection:
  ◆ Prep and drape the digit (or entire hand) sterilely.
  ◆ Administer digital anaesthetic (see Appendix B).
  ◆ A digital tourniquet using a penrose drain, or the finger from a sterile glove, can help control bleeding.
  ◆ Make a mid-lateral incision (see Figure 23-1); do not incise the volar pulp because it can lead to a tender scar.
  ◆ Insert a hemostat through the incision perpendicular and palmar to the distal phalanx; open hemostat inside pulp to break apart septa and allow drainage of pus. Try not to enter the area of the flexor tendon insertion and risk seeding the flexor tendon sheath.
  ◆ Send specimen for Gram stain, culture (aerobic and anaerobic, atypical mycobacteria, and fungus, if suspected because of patient's activities or chronicity), and sensitivity if there is a specimen. Do not swab the skin, or the culture will grow many skin flora.
  ◆ Irrigate the wound thoroughly with normal saline and pack with sterile packing gauze to facilitate drainage.
  ◆ Dress with sterile dressings.

# COLOR ATLAS

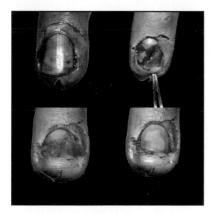

**Figure 5-3.** This crush injury resulted in a distal phalanx fracture with considerable subungual hematoma. Removal of the nail plate revealed a large nail bed laceration. This was repaired with 6-0 chromic suture. The nail plate was replaced under the eponychial fold; if the nail plate is not available, foil (such as from a suture package) may be inserted instead. *Also shown on page 28.*

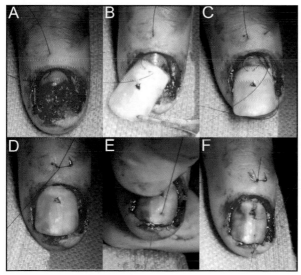

**Figure 5-4.** The nail plate is replaced beneath the eponychial fold and sutured as shown with 5-0 nylon to prevent dislodgement (A-D). An additional suture through the nail plate into the hyponychium (E-F) secures the plate to the nail bed. Note drainage hole placed in nail plate with blade. *Also shown on page 29.*

CA-1

**Figure 23-1.** Felon infection with erythema and subcutaneous abscess; a mid-lateral incision allows insertion of a hemostat to evacuate septal compartments. (Photo courtesy of Dr. Jeffrey C. King.) *Also shown on page 110.*

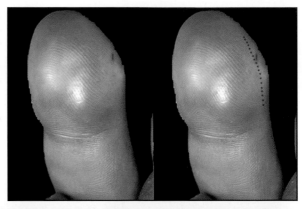

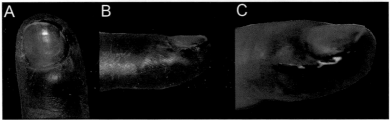

**Figure 24-1.** This patient presented with a paronychial infection exhibiting erythema as well as a fluctuant lateral abscess (A and B). A lateral incision along the paronychial fold relieved the pressure; irrigation, soaks, and antibiotics led to resolution. *Also shown on page 115.*

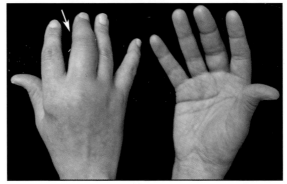

**Figure 25-1.** This patient presented with a 1-day history of right long finger swelling, pain, and redness. Examination demonstrated Kanavel signs: a swollen "sausage-like" digit, a flexed resting posture, tenderness to palpation along the flexor sheath, and pain with passive extension of the digit. Early diagnosis and inpatient treatment with intravenous antibiotics, splinting, soaks, and strict elevation resulted in resolution without surgical intervention. *Also shown on page 118.*

**Figure 27-1.** This patient developed a web space infection around his ring finger likely related to his psoriatic lesions; the puncture wounds were self-inflicted to "drain the pressure" when the purulence started tracking distally into the digit. *Also shown on page 126.*

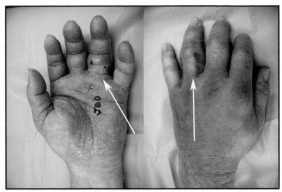

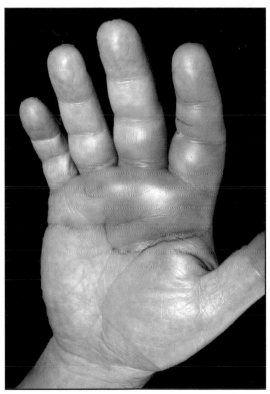

**Figure 28-1.** This patient developed painful erythema without inciting event. He was admitted to the hospital and the cellulitis resolved with empiric IV antibiotic treatment, splinting, and elevation. *Also shown on page 130.*

- Start oral antibiotics after obtaining culture; empiric treatment for *S. aureus* is indicated until cultures or lack of clinical improvement demonstrate otherwise.
- Referral to hand surgeon within 48 hours.

## Definitive Treatment (Refer to Hand Specialist)

- Most felons resolve following a regimen of soaks and dressing changes, and a course of antibiotics, but the wound must be monitored closely.
- Repeat incision and drainage sometimes is necessary if reaccumulation occurs.
- The wound heals by secondary intention and generally leaves a cosmetically acceptable scar.

## Potential Problems

- Scar tenderness can develop, and can be a problem, if the incision is located on the volar pulp of the digit.
- Recurrence of infection, or persistent infection, can result in osteomyelitis.
- Digits become stiff with prolonged immobilization; range of motion exercises, rather than splinting, are encouraged.

### SUGGESTED READING

Abrams RA, Botte MJ. Hand infections: treatment recommendations for specific types. *J Am Acad Orthop Surg*. 1996;4:219-230.

Connolly B, Johnstone F, Gerlinger T, Puttler E. Methicillin-resistant Staphylococcus aureus in a finger felon. *J Hand Surg [Am]*. 2000;25(1):173-175.

Jebson PJ. Infections of the fingertip. Paronychias and felons. *Hand Clin*. 1998;14(4):547-555.

# chapter 24

# PARONYCHIAL INFECTIONS

Paronychial infections, or infections of the soft tissues surrounding the nail plate, are common in patients who get manicures, have artificial nails, bite their nails, or have hangnails. The most common organism causing acute infections is *S. aureus*. Chronic paronychial infections usually are found in those whose digits are constantly exposed to moisture in their occupation. These chronic infections usually involve fungus, atypical mycobacterium, or Gram negative organisms.

## Mechanism of Injury

- The patient usually is inoculated through the skin, and an abscess develops between the nail plate and the eponychial fold; the infection spreads between the nail plate and the eponychial or peronychial area.
- Chronic paronychial infection is common in patients whose occupations involve continuous water exposure (eg, dishwashers).

## Evaluation

- Patient complains of tenderness, swelling, redness, or even drainage around the nail plate.
- Ask the patient about any recent exposures to manicure instruments, artificial nails, nailbiting, or hangnails. Also inquire about chronic moisture exposure, either occupationally or during pursuit of hobbies.

- Examination of acute infection reveals swollen, erythematous, tender abscess—with or without purulent drainage—next to the nail plate (Figure 24-1).
- Evaluate for puncture wound or other possible source.
- "Lifting" of the eponychium from the nail plate, or "cheesy" discharge, can indicate a chronic infection.

## Acute Treatment

- Chronic infections do not need to be treated acutely; they should be referred to a hand surgeon for management.
- Acute infections demonstrating only cellulitis can be treated with antibiotics.
- If an abscess is present, this must be drained:
  - Prep and drape digit (or entire hand) sterilely.
  - Administer digital anaesthetic block.
  - If the abscess extends to the nail plate, sometimes it can drain by inserting Freer elevator or #15 blade between the nail plate and eponychium.
  - If necessary, incise along the paronychium/eponychium, but do not violate the nail bed or a nail deformity will result (see Figure 24-1).
  - If purulent drainage occurs, send specimen for Gram stain, culture, and sensitivity (aerobic, anaerobic, atypicals, and fungals if suspected because of patient activities or chronicity of infection).
  - Irrigate with sterile saline, place sterile wick in wound, and apply sterile dressing.
  - Administer antibiotics after obtaining cultures; the usual organism is *S. aureus.*
  - Refer to hand surgeon for evaluation within days.

## Definitive Treatment (Refer to Hand Specialist)

- Ensure adequate drainage and no reaccumulation of abscess.
- Soaks will be recommended per hand surgeon preference.
- Oral antibiotics are used to treat the infection.

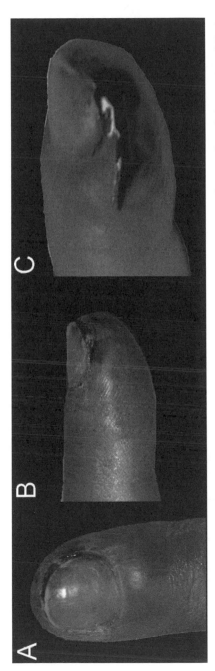

**Figure 24-1.** This patient presented with a paronychial infection exhibiting erythema as well as a fluctuant lateral abscess (A and B). A lateral incision along the paronychial fold relieved the pressure; irrigation, soaks, and antibiotics led to resolution. *For a full-color version, see page CA-II of the Color Atlas.*

- Chronic infections often are best treated operatively by "marsupialization," or excision of part of the eponychium and nail plate removal.

## Potential Problems

- Infection can spread and create felon or purulent tenosynovitis.
- Damage to the nail bed can occur and create nail plate deformity.

### SUGGESTED READING

Abrams RA, Botte MJ. Hand infections: treatment recommendations for specific types. *J Am Acad Orthop Surg.* 1996;4(4):219-230.

Jebson PJ. Infections of the fingertip. Paronychias and felons. *Hand Clin.* 1998;14(4):547-555.

Yates YJ, Concannon MJ. Fungal infections of the perionychium. *Hand Clin.* 2002;18(4):631-642.

# chapter 25

# INFECTIOUS/PURULENT TENOSYNOVITIS

Infectious tenosynovitis is an infection in the synovial sheath surrounding the flexor tendon. Usually, the index, long, and ring digits have their own sheaths, extending from the tip of the digit to the distal palmar crease. The sheath of the small digit extends from the tip of the digit proximally into the "ulnar bursa." The thumb flexor sheath extends proximally to the "radial bursa." Communication of the radial and ulnar bursae can result in a "horseshoe abscess" at the level of the wrist.

## Mechanism of Injury

- The patient might recall a penetrating injury (bite, thorn, laceration).
- Sometimes, there is no history of injury; hematogenous spread (especially of an organism like *Neisseria gonorrhoeae*) is possible.

## Evaluation

- Determine if the patient has any risk factors for exposure (penetrating injury) or progressive infection (diabetes, immunocompromise).
- Identify any puncture wounds or other potential source of infection.
- Examine digit for 4 Kanavel signs: 1) flexed resting posture, 2) sausage-like swelling, 3) tenderness of flexor tendon sheath, and, most commonly, 4) pain with passive extension of the digit (Figure 25-1).

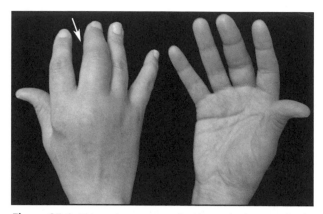

**Figure 25-1.** This patient presented with a 1-day history of right long finger swelling, pain, and redness. Examination demonstrated Kanavel signs: a swollen "sausage-like" digit, a flexed resting posture, tenderness to palpation along the flexor sheath, and pain with passive extension of the digit. Early diagnosis and inpatient treatment with intravenous antibiotics, splinting, soaks, and strict elevation resulted in resolution without surgical intervention. *For a full-color version, see page CA-II of the Color Atlas.*

- Radiographs might show a foreign body. Ultrasound sometimes can identify small retained foreign bodies (eg, 3-mm segment of thorn), or fluid collection in or around the tendon sheath; ultrasound, however, might be poorly tolerated in the setting of purulent tenosynovitis.
- Obtain basic laboratory studies: complete blood count (CBC), glucose, erythrocyte sedimentation rate (ESR), and C-reactive protein (CRP). If patient is febrile, send blood culture.

## Acute Treatment

- True purulent flexor tenosynovitis is a surgical emergency and, therefore, a hand surgery consult is warranted if there is suspicion.
- Mild or early symptoms can be treated with IV antibiotics, splinting, and strict elevation; this might lead to resolution.

## Definitive Treatment (Refer to Hand Specialist)

- Urgent surgical irrigation and debridement to eradicate infection is performed if there is purulence.
- The patient is treated as an inpatient with IV antibiotics, splinting, and elevation until infection is resolving.
- Repeat irrigation and debridement might be required.

## Potential Problems

- Loss of digit or function of the digit due to tendon necrosis or scarring.
- Infections can spread to palm, other digits, or systemically.

*SUGGESTED READING*

Abrams RA, Botte MJ. Hand infections: treatment recommendations for specific types. *J Am Acad Orthop Surg.* 1996;4(4):219-230.

Boles SC, Schmidt CC. Pyogenic flexor tenosynovitis. *Hand Clin.* 1998;14(4):567-578.

# chapter 26

## SEPTIC ARTHRITIS

Septic arthritis, or infection of the joint, is a surgical emergency. Exposure of an articular surface to the acute inflammatory response and to bacterial toxins results in degradation of cartilage relatively quickly with potentially devastating results. Prompt recognition, differentiation from inflammatory arthritis (especially gout or pseudogout), and appropriate treatment are critical.

## Mechanism of Injury

- Joints can become seeded with bacteria from the outside (puncture wound, eg, thorn) or the inside (bacteremia, eg, endocarditis).
- Even though non-native joints (replacements) do not have cartilage, infection causes a coating to form on the implant; infection of a joint replacement might require even more extensive surgery than infection of a native joint.

## Evaluation

- Patient might complain of erythema, swelling, and pain around affected joint.
- In a native joint, minimal range of motion of joint can cause severe pain or even be intolerable.
- Particularly in the hand and wrist, gout or pseudogout can mimic a septic joint; a definitive diagnosis is needed to rule out (or rule in) infection.
- Radiographs often are normal, but can show widening of the joint space, erosion of the joint surface, or deposition disease (most commonly associated with pseudogout).

- Laboratory values: CBC, glucose, ESR, CRP, urate (can be elevated in gout attack), and blood cultures should be sent.
- Prior to any antibiotic administration, an aspirate should be obtained sterilely and preferably not through an area of cellulitis/erythema (consult hand surgeon if you are not comfortable with this) and sent for:
  - Cell count: will determine the likelihood of septic versus inflammatory condition. Often, the WBC in an aspirate from a septic joint can be in excess of 100,000.
  - Gram stain: unlikely to show organisms unless floridly infected.
  - Culture and sensitivity: will help determine appropriate antibiotic treatment regimen; if atypical mycobacterium or fungus is suspected, inform the microbiology lab when sending the culture so that special tests can be performed.
  - Crystals can be indicative of gout or pseudogout.

## Acute Treatment

- Septic arthritis destroys cartilage and is a surgical emergency; a hand surgeon should be consulted immediately for evaluation.
- Preoperative preparation is helpful.
- Keep patient NPO in case of need for surgical intervention.
- Do not start antibiotics until a specimen has been obtained and sent for culture.
- The most common organisms are *Staphylococcus aureus* and streptococci. In children younger than 6 months, *S. aureus* and gram-negative anaerobes are most common. In children aged 6 months to 2 years, *S. aureus* and *Haemophilus influenzae* are the usual organisms. Suspect *Neisseria gonorrhoeae* in those who are, or might be, sexually active.

## Definitive Treatment (Refer to Hand Specialist)

- Irrigation and debridement is performed urgently.
- The course of antibiotic treatment depends upon organism and patient characteristics.
- Patient might need additional surgeries depending on extent of damage and ability to control and eradicate infection.

## Potential Problems

- Spread or persistence of infection can be a problem.
- Cartilage destruction leading to chronic painful arthritis or joint dysfunction can occur.
- Stiffness or loss of function might result.

### SUGGESTED READING

Abrams RA, Botte MJ. Hand infections: treatment recommendations for specific types. *J Am Acad Orthop Surg.* 1996;4(4):219-230.

Murray PM. Septic arthritis of the hand and wrist. *Hand Clin.* 1998;14(4):579-587.

# chapter 27

# WEB SPACE INFECTION (COLLAR-BUTTON ABSCESS) AND PALMAR SPACE INFECTIONS

The hand has several "deep spaces" that can allow for spread of infection and confinement within a discrete area. The concepts of the ulnar and radial bursae are addressed in Chapter 25. Web space infections that develop between the digits and can spread into the palm are discussed here.

## Mechanism of Injury

- These can originate from puncture wounds, blisters, psoriatic lesions, or callouses.
- The infection spreads dorsally and palmarly in the web space and can spread through palmar spaces.

## Evaluation

- Inquire about history of wounds, exposure to infection, fever, chills, or other systemic symptoms.
- Inspect for swelling, erythema, and wounds; digits might be "held apart" by web space infection (Figure 27-1).
- Palpate for tenderness, fluctuant areas, and lymphadenopathy.
- Relevant laboratory studies: order CBC with differential, ESR, and CRP. If patient febrile, blood cultures should be sent.
- Radiographs can be used to assess for radiopaque foreign body or fracture (often confused with infection in diabetic patients).

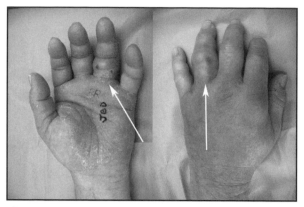

**Figure 27-1.** This patient developed a web space infection around his ring finger likely related to his psoriatic lesions. The puncture wounds were self-inflicted to "drain the pressure" when the purulence started tracking distally into the digit. *For a full-color version, see page CA-III of the Color Atlas.*

## Acute Treatment

- Provide pain management. Splint for comfort with a volar plaster splint and elevate the hand.
- Keep patient NPO for possible surgery.
- Consult hand surgeon immediately for consideration of surgical incision and drainage (I&D).
- Do not administer antibiotics prior to adequate intraoperative culture; this can invalidate culture results and complicate the treatment course.

## Definitive Treatment (Refer to Hand Specialist)

- Surgical I&D with or without catheter irrigation is likely.
- The required antibiotic course can range from days to weeks.

## Potential Problems

- Inadequate treatment (surgically or pharmacologically) can lead to continued or spread of infection, resulting in stiffness, deformity, and loss of function.

## SUGGESTED READING

Abrams RA, Botte MJ. Hand infections: treatment recommendations for specific types. *J Am Acad Orthop Surg.* 1996;4(4):219-230.

# chapter 28

# CELLULITIS

Cellulitis is a bacterial infection of the skin which, if left untreated, can result in spread of infection, formation of abscess (or infectious tenosynovitis), or other serious consequences. In general, this can be managed nonoperatively if caught before any collections develop. An important differential diagnosis is necrotizing fasciitis, which is a limb- and potentially life-threatening surgical emergency.

## Mechanism of Injury

- The patient might recall a puncture wound, insect bite, or scratch on digit or extremity.
- Superficial skin infection can spread proximally up the arm.

## Evaluation

- Determine patient and environmental risk factors (diabetic, exposure to organisms, history of trauma in affected area).
- Assess erythema, swelling, warmth, and tenderness of skin and subcutaneous tissues (Figure 28-1).
- Must differentiate from septic joint; cellulitis is painful superficially, not necessarily with joint motion. Must also differentiate from necrotizing fasciitis, which is very painful, rapidly progressive, and usually associated with more systemic symptoms (acute illness is much more "impressive" than the early skin changes).
- Identify any skin lesions from which infection might have originated.

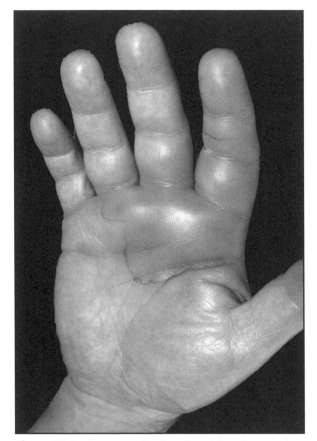

**Figure 28-1.** This patient developed painful erythema without inciting event. He was admitted to the hospital and the cellulitis resolved with empiric IV antibiotic treatment, splinting, and elevation. *For a full-color version, see page CA-III of the Color Atlas.*

- Assess for red "streaking" up arm due to lymphangitis and adenopathy, indicative of potential systemic spreading.
- Assess radiographs for free air from *Clostridium* infection.
- Labs: CBC looking for an elevated WBC, glucose (diabetic?), ESR, CRP to monitor infection.
- If febrile or systemically ill, obtain blood cultures to determine bacteremia.

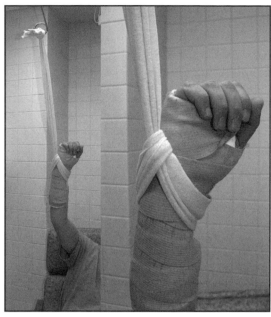

**Figure 28-2.** "Strict elevation" is accomplished by using a stockinette gently looped around the splint and attached to an IV pole or ceiling fixture (as shown). Placing the hand on a pillow generally is too short term and rarely creates enough elevation.

## Acute Treatment

- Have a low threshold for admitting patient to hospital for observation.
- Start empiric IV antibiotics: ampicillin/sulbactam is usually the first-line intravenous agent.
- Splint hand/wrist in neutral position for comfort and elevate from IV pole or ceiling fixture (Figure 28-2).
- Consult hand surgeon if there is a question of abscess, infectious tenosynovitis, septic joint, or necrotizing fasciitis.

## Definitive Treatment (Refer to Hand Specialist)

- Cellulitis is treated nonoperatively, but hand surgeons will differentiate cellulitis from an abscess, septic joint, purulent flexor tenosynovitis, or other surgical emergencies.

## Potential Problems

- Infection can spread locally or systemically.
- Soft tissue damage might lead to stiffness or other loss of function.

### SUGGESTED READING

Abrams RA, Botte MJ. Hand infections: treatment recommendations for specific types. *J Am Acad Orthop Surg.* 1996;4(4):219-230.

# chapter 29

## *HERPETIC WHITLOW*

Herpetic whitlow has an annual incidence of 2.5 to 5 cases per 100,000 people. This condition generally resolves spontaneously, but misdiagnosis as a paronychial infection with subsequent incision can lead to bacterial infection or viral spread. Consider this before incising a paronychial infection, especially in a health care worker or immunocompromised patient.

### Mechanism of Injury

- Patient is inoculated with herpes simplex virus (HSV) 1 or 2 in an area of broken skin.
- Health care workers or others exposed to oral or genital herpes are at risk.

### Evaluation

- Identify any risk factors (occupational or other exposure).
- Assess for erythema, edema, or tenderness; these lesions often are quite painful. Early stages can show the clear vesicles of HSV 1 or 2, while later stages can look like a bacterial infection.
- Evaluate patient for fever or lymphadenopathy.
- Tzanck test, viral culture, or DNA testing can confirm diagnosis.

## Acute Treatment

- If patient presents within 48 hours of onset, valacyclovir, acyclovir, or famciclovir might be helpful.
- Advise patient to cover the lesion with a dry dressing to prevent spreading of the virus.
- Do not incise the lesion. This can cause systemic viremia or cause a secondary bacterial infection.
- Reassure the patient that the lesion should resolve on its own within a few weeks, although it can recur.

## Definitive Treatment (Refer to Hand Specialist)

- A hand surgeon who identifies this as herpetic whitlow will reassure the patient (as above) that operating on this will worsen the condition.

## Potential Problems

- The virus can spread locally or systemically and can be spread to others.
- Incision of the lesion can cause worsening of the infection and secondary bacterial infection.
- Recurrence is noted 30% to 50% of the time, although usually with less severe symptoms.

### SUGGESTED READING

Fowler JR. Viral infections. *Hand Clin.* 1989;5(4):613-627.
Wu IB, Schwartz RA. Herpetic whitlow. *Cutis.* 2007;79:193-196.

# chapter 30

## BITE WOUNDS

Bite wounds often are much more serious than they appear at first glance. The most common bites are from dogs, cats, or humans. It is estimated that 3.5 million to 4.7 million domestic animal bites occur every year in the United States.[1] According to the same group, two-thirds of patients required hospital admission for at least IV antibiotics, and one-third had undergone at least one surgery following a cat or dog bite. Patzakis et al found that 75% of patients with "fight bites" (clenched-fist injuries in which a human tooth caused a puncture) had tendon, joint, cartilage, or bone damage.[2] These bites need to be evaluated and treated early, and relatively aggressively, to prevent infection, identify and repair injured structures, and prevent short- and long-term complications.

### Mechanism of Injury

- Most animal bites result from either a patient trying to separate 2 fighting animals or attempting to help a sick animal.
- Dog bites create extensive soft tissue damage because of tearing.
- Cat bites generally are puncture wounds, but more prone to infection than dog bites.
- Fight bites from fist to mouth can result in MCP joint penetration by a tooth.

### Evaluation

- Examine wounds; document location, size, and degree of observable soft tissue damage.

- Identify involved structures, including penetration into joints and tendon, nerve, and blood vessel injuries. Remember to consider the anatomy present around that area and "test" those structures accordingly.
- Keep in mind that the location, size, and number of wounds have not been found to correlate with the severity of morbidity associated with the bite(s) and should not be used as criteria for treatment decisions. However, bite wounds that involve closed spaces (joints, pulp of fingertip, flexor tendon sheath) are predisposed to infection and more likely to require surgery and an extended course of antibiotics.
- Assess radiographs for fracture, foreign body (tooth), or air in joint space, indicating that the joint has been penetrated.

## Acute Treatment

- Administer rabies immune globulin and/or vaccine, if indicated (Appendix D).
- Irrigate and debride wounds. Cat bite puncture wounds tend to close relatively quickly; they should be opened and allowed to drain.
- Similarly, resist the urge to suture dog bite lacerations; they need to drain.
- IV ampicillin/sulbactam, or can use clindamycin if allergic to penicillin; IV ertapenem is becoming popular as it is dosed daily (not every 6 hours).
- If the wound is fresh (<6 hours) and the patient is reliable, you might be able to administer a single IV dose of ampicillin/sulbactam and discharge on oral amoxicillin/clavulanic acid.
- Maintain a low threshold for admission, IV antibiotics, elevation, and observation, particularly in pediatric, geriatric, and diabetic patients.
- Patient should be instructed about importance of compliance with elevation, antibiotics, and follow-up to prevent infection and disability.

## Definitive Treatment (Refer to Hand Specialist)

- Patients should follow up within 24 to 48 hours to limit chances of progressive infection and promote appropriate aftercare.
- Operative intervention is indicated for open joints, deep infection, frank purulence, tendon or neurovascular injury, or potential fracture.
- Antibiotics and intermittent debridement might be needed.
- Hand therapy can be prescribed to assist with wound care, decrease swelling, and improve range of motion.

## Potential Problems

- Infection, including tenosynovitis, cellulitis, septic arthritis, or osteomyelitis, can occur.
- Stiffness, or other loss of function due to edema, scarring, or delay in treatment
- Pain

### REFERENCES

1. Benson LS, Edwards SL, Schiff AP, Williams CS, Visotsky JI. Dog and cat bites to the hand: treatment and cost assessment. *J Hand Surg [Am]*. 2006;31(3):468-473.
2. Patzakis MJ, Wilkins J, Bassett RL. Surgical findings in clenched-fist injuries. *Clin Orthop Relat Res*. 1987;220:237-240.

### SUGGESTED READING

Chuinard RG, D'Ambrosia RD. Human bite infections in the hand. *J Bone Joint Surg Am*. 1977;59(3):416-418.
Murray PM. Septic arthritis of the hand and wrist. *Hand Clin*. 1998;14(4):579-587.

# Section VI

## Other Traumatic Digit Injuries

# chapter 31

# *TRAUMATIC AMPUTATIONS*

Traumatic amputations can be frightening for both patients and providers. Since "replantation" became feasible with microsurgical advancements, there has evolved a general assumption that any part brought in with the patient can, and should, be reattached. However, replantation is complicated and is performed at a limited number of facilities equipped not only with hand surgeons, but with the appropriate support team. Short- and long-term failures associated with replants have resulted in the following indications for replanting digits:

1.    Any digit in a child
2.    Multiple digits in adults
3.    Thumb amputation

It is best to complete the evaluation and discuss treatment with a hand surgeon before promising a patient that a digit can be replanted. More often than not, completion amputation results in a more functional, cosmetically acceptable hand with earlier return to activity than replantation.

A meta-analysis in 2006 by Dec[1] showed poor prognostic factors for replantation to include those associated with the patient (smoking, diabetes, male gender), injury pattern (crush or avulsion), level of amputation (distal phalanx, thumb IP joint or distal), and presentation (delay of 12 hours).

## Mechanism of Injury

- Clean cut (saw, knife, guillotine)
- Crush (greater zone of injury)
- Avulsion (tendons, nerves, vessels get "pulled out" with the digit)

## Evaluation

- Determine patient factors that might influence decision making: age, hand dominance, occupation, avocation, and medical comorbidities.
- Ask about injury mechanism, and particularly about how long ago this happened.
- Evaluate level and mechanism of amputation.
- If incomplete, assess vascular status of digit.
- Assess radiographs of hand and amputated digit(s) (if present) to determine extent of bone and joint involvement.

## Acute Treatment

- Urgent treatment includes tetanus prophylaxis, IV antibiotics, and pain control.
- If available, wrap the amputated digit in saline-moistened gauze and place in plastic bag; the bag can be placed on ice (do not place amputated digit directly on ice or soak in saline).
- Contact hand surgeon immediately to discuss whether replantation is feasible.
- If replantation is reasonable, start preparations for transfer to the operating room or transfer to a facility where replantation is performed.
- If not, discuss with hand surgeon further treatment (emergency room irrigation, closure, and referral versus hand surgeon coming to treat patient).

## Potential Problems

- Infection
- Loss of function (stiffness due to tendon adhesions/scarring, sensory deficit)
- Pain, especially due to cold intolerance
- Atrophy of the digits due to poor circulation

## REFERENCE

1. Dec W. A meta-analysis of success rates for digit replantation. *Tech Hand Up Extrem Surg.* 2006;10(3):124-129.

## SUGGESTED READING

Soucacos PN. Indications and selection for digital amputation and replantation. *J Hand Surg [Br].* 2001;26(6):572-581.

chapter $32$

# INJECTION INJURIES

High-pressure injection injuries can be deceptively benign in presentation, but if not identified immediately and treated surgically, catastrophe can result. The outcome of such an injury depends on what was injected, amount of material, pressure at which material was injected, and length of time between injury and surgery.

## Mechanism of Injury

- Injection usually occurs while the patient is cleaning an injection nozzle, therefore, the injury often affects the index finger of the nondominant hand.
- Nozzle pressures are very high, so contact between skin and nozzle is not necessary for a person to sustain a serious injury.
- Paint solvents cause inflammation, while grease produces chronic fibrosis.

## Evaluation

- Determine how the injury happened, when, what was injected, and approximately how much material.
- Patient might complain of burning, numbness, or pain.
- Wound may appear benign (like a small puncture wound) even with significant soft tissue damage.
- Assess for crepitation in the soft tissues, which suggests subcutaneous air.
- Injections at IP joint creases can penetrate the flexor tendon sheath and result in spreading throughout the palmar spaces;

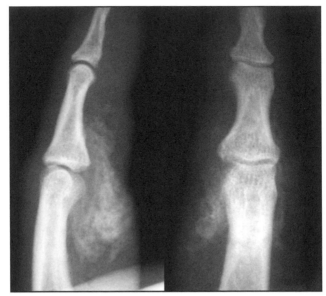

**Figure 32-1.** Radiographs of this digit show radiopacity of injected latex material. (Radiograph courtesy of Dr. Fraser J. Leversedge.)

injections between these creases usually result in more superficial wounds.

- Radiopaque substances or free air can be localized using radiographs (Figure 32-1).

## Acute Treatment

- Start IV antibiotics to include a first-generation cephalosporin and an aminoglycoside to prevent secondary infection.
- Liver function, blood urea nitrogen (BUN), and creatinine should be monitored because some injectables are toxic to the liver and cause hematuria.
- Consult a hand surgeon immediately for evaluation and management.

## Definitive Treatment (Refer to Hand Specialist)

- Urgent surgical debridement (preferably within 6 hours of injury) might be required.

- Neurovascular injury and tissue necrosis can be severe enough to necessitate amputation.

## Potential Problems

- Neurovascular injury, necrosis, fibrosis, or infection can necessitate amputation.
- Secondary infection can occur.

### SUGGESTED READING

American College of Emergency Physicians. Clinical policy for the initial approach to patients presenting with penetrating extremity trauma. *Ann Emerg Med.* 1999;33(5):612-636.

Stengel D, Bauwens K, Sehouli J, Ekkernkamp A, Porzsolt F. Systematic review and meta-analysis of antibiotic therapy for bone and joint infections. *Lancet Infect Dis.* 2001;1(3):175-188.

# chapter 33

# RING AVULSION INJURIES

Injury to the ring finger from a ring avulsion is not only problematic cosmetically, the function and sensibility of the ring finger are important for gripping and holding objects. These injuries range from superficial soft tissue injuries to complete degloving of the soft tissue from bone.

## Mechanism of Injury

- The ring catches on a hook, basketball net, or another object and strangulates the finger; or the ring is too tight because of swelling (Figure 33-1).
- The same type of injury can be caused if the finger is caught by a string or rope (eg, sailing).
- Classification is based on vascular damage:
  - Class I: adequate circulation
  - Class II: inadequate circulation (requires vascular repair)
  - Class III: complete degloving (requires replantation)

## Evaluation

- If the ring is still present, remove it (Appendix E).
- Determine whether there is compromised perfusion:
  - Capillary refill
  - Digital Allen test
  - Doppler digital vessels
- Recognize that digital vessel disruption can occur, even without skin laceration.

149

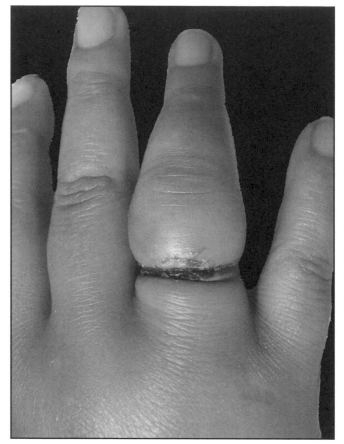

**Figure 33-1.** This edematous digit was strangulated by a ring left in place following an injury. (Photo courtesy of Dr. Fraser J. Leversedge.)

- Assess extent and location of additional soft tissue injury (nerves, vessels, tendons, bone).
- Radiographs: AP, lateral, and oblique radiographs of the digit are needed to determine whether a fracture, dislocation, or subluxation occurred.

## Acute Treatment

- Keep the digit warm with gentle irrigation of the wound and wrap it in gauze soaked in warm saline.

- Do not ligate or cauterize digital vessels before speaking with a hand surgeon; this will hinder microvascular repair.
- Even if the injury is Class I, leave the skin laceration open to prevent constriction of blood vessels.

## Definitive Treatment (Refer to Hand Specialist)

- These injuries are often worse than they appear. Even if circulation appears to be adequate, arterial thrombosis and progressive ischemia is possible, and the patient should be seen by a hand surgeon as soon as possible for complete evaluation.
- If perfusion is compromised (or there is any question of it), call a hand surgeon immediately; this may require urgent vascular repair.

## Potential Problems

- Progressive ischemia from vascular disruption can necessitate amputation.
- Even with urgent surgical treatment, patients might have altered sensation (paresthesias, hyperesthesias) or motion (tendon scarring, joint fusion, skin contracture).

*SUGGESTED READING*

Kay S, Werntz J, Wolff TW. Ring avulsion injuries: classification and prognosis. *J Hand Surg [Am]*. 1989;14(2 Pt 1):204-213.

Urbaniak JR, Evans JP, Bright DS. Microvascular management of ring avulsion injuries. *J Hand Surg [Am]*. 1981;6(1):25-30.

# Section VII

## Gunshot Wounds, Burns, and Frostbite

# chapter 34

# GUNSHOT WOUNDS

Because of the compact tissue volumes and intricate anatomy in the hand, gunshot wounds to the hand can cause devastating injuries. Often, multiple structures are injured, and the treatment is complicated by balancing a need for immobilization of some injuries (eg, fractures), with a need for early motion of others (eg, tendon repairs). Thorough assessment of potentially injured structures and appropriate initial treatment are the goals of the acute management period.

## Mechanism of Injury

- Gunshot wounds cause tissue damage because of both penetration and blast injury.
- Extent of damage is proportional to energy of injury: small handguns or BB guns are "low energy," while rifles and larger caliber handguns are "high energy" and tend to cause more damage.
- Shotguns disperse pellets and other debris, and usually cause the worst injuries.

## Evaluation

- Determine entry and exit sites of bullet, and use possible trajectory to anticipate structures that might have been injured (Figure 34-1).
- Note areas of skin loss or laceration.
- A thorough exam will help identify vascular compromise (do not miss a palmar arch or other vessel injury), tendon injuries, or nerve deficits.

**Figure 34-1.** Gunshot wound to the lateral arm created a large soft tissue injury and multiple fractures. Evaluation of the location of the entry wound and the radiographs allow one to predict that this patient might have a radial nerve palsy, which he did. Subsequent treatment involved I&D, stabilization of the fractures, nerve exploration (the radial nerve injury was blast, not laceration), and removal of the large bullet fragments.

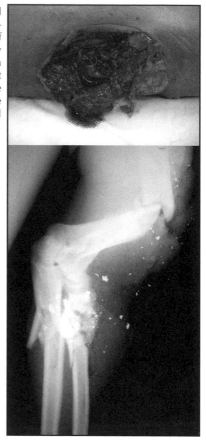

- Blast injury can cause nerve dysfunction far from the site of the bullet, particularly in a small space like the hand, so assess each nerve by checking if every motor and sensory function is preserved.
- Radiographs of the sites of injury are needed to identify fractures (see Figure 34-1).

## Acute Treatment

- Administer antibiotics and tetanus (if needed).
- Irrigate wound with warm saline.

- Monitor clinically for compartment syndrome while patient is under your care.
- Contact hand surgeon to determine timing of treatment; if there is going to be any delay in evaluation, cover wound with non-adherent dressing and apply well-padded volar and dorsal plaster splints with MCP joints flexed and wrist slightly extended.

## Definitive Treatment (Refer to Hand Specialist)

- A quick phone call to the surgeon will aid in determining timing for definitive treatment.
- Surgical management can include wound care, fracture treatment, tendon, nerve, and/or vessel repair, fasciotomies, soft tissue coverage, etc, depending upon the extent of the injury.
- Even if the patient seems very lucky in that everything seems intact, it is best to refer for specialist evaluation so that nothing is missed. Many such patients will benefit from a course of splinting and hand therapy.

## Potential Problems

- Blast injury can lead to phantom pain and complex regional pain syndrome.
- Patients should be warned that further procedures like skin grafts, flaps, or even amputation might be needed to manage the injury. Patients also must understand that loss of motion or sensation, infection, and pain all are potential complications associated with this injury.

*Suggested Reading*

Al-Qattan MM. Air gun pellet injuries of the hand. *J Hand Surg [Br]*. 2006;31(2):178-181.

Wilson RH. Gunshots to the hand and upper extremity. *Clin Orthop Relat Res*. 2003;(408):133-144.

# chapter 35

# BURNS

Burns cause some of the most severe hand injuries. Because of the compact anatomy and the necessity for gliding of many hand structures, the hand is extremely sensitive to burn injury and terrible functional deficits can occur with improper care. Experience in management of burn injuries is important and, if necessary, patients should be transferred to an appropriate facility equipped to stabilize and treat burn victims.

## Evaluation

Patients with burns of the hand should be treated as trauma patients. Full evaluation and management of the most emergent issues (airway, breathing, circulation, smoke inhalation, fluid resuscitation) takes priority. When assessing the burn, it is important to determine:

- The nature of exposure—electrical, flame, flash, tar/asphalt, scale, chemical, steam, and grease all can cause burns and treatment options vary depending on etiology.
- Length of time exposed
- Percentage of body surface area affected (palmar surface of the hand is considered 1%, a single upper extremity is 9%)
- Location of the burn: dorsal skin is thinner than volar skin
- Degree of burn:
  - First degree: red area, superficial
  - Second degree: dermal, blisters, possible unroofing of raw reddish area
  - Third degree: full thickness, can be insensate, leathery
  - Fourth degree: involving tendon, bone, or other deeper structures

- Assess for vascular compromise, remembering that hypovolemia from under-resuscitation can result in absent pulses; in an adequately hydrated patient with circumferential burns, however, an absent pulse might be an indication for escharotomy (surgery).

## Acute Treatment

- Administer tetanus prophylaxis.
- If the burn is entirely superficial (erythema only), it can be treated with moisturization and immediate mobilization.
- Superficial partial-thickness burns can be treated with bacitracin ointment and nonadherent dressings.
- Deep dermal burns should be treated twice daily with 1% Silver sulfadiazine cream and nonadherent and dry dressings.
- Early mobilization, elevation, and pain control are key for all burn wounds.

## Definitive Treatment (Refer to Hand Specialist)

- Outpatients should be evaluated by a hand surgeon within approximately 48 hours for wound care, and determination of surgical and rehabilitation needs.
- Severe wounds might require surgery, including escharotomy, fasciotomy, debridements, skin grafts, or flaps, in addition to addressing any other damaged structures.

## Potential Problems

- Compartment syndrome
- Contractures
- Syndactyly
- Infections

## *Special Consideration: Chemical Burns*

Chemical burns can be deceptive because of the chemical agent's inherent ability to stay in solution instead of precipitate. Alkali chemicals in particular can continue to cause tissue necrosis until neutralized appropriately. It therefore is very important to determine the exact cause of the burn, duration of exposure (which persists until the agent is removed or neutralized), and pre-evaluation treatment, and identify and administer the correct antidote. For a table of common agents causing chemical burns and basic management guidelines, see Appendix G.

## Acute Treatment

- Remove any clothing contaminated with the agent.
- Irrigate the burn area with copious amounts of water, unless the burning agent is elemental sodium, potassium, or lithium. These agents can ignite if they are exposed to water.
- Hydrofluoric acid (rust removers):
    - Check serum $Ca^{2+}$.
    - 2.5% calcium gluconate gel
    - Large burns might require neutralization with 10% calcium gluconate injected subcutaneously, 0.5 cc/cm$^2$.
    - If >2% of body surface area is burned, inject a solution of 2 g calcium gluconate in 250 cc dextrose 5% in water over 4 hours via radial arterial line (with cardiac monitoring).
- Hydrochloric acid (pool cleaners): magnesium oxide and soap
- Organics (petroleum solvents): dilute soap and water.

### Special Consideration: Electrical Burns

Electrical burns can result from household (low-voltage) or industrial (high-voltage) accidents; in either circumstance, clothing can ignite. The current passes from an entrance wound to an exit wound, so considerable soft tissue injury can result throughout the body.

High-voltage injuries are very serious. Patients should be admitted to a trauma or burn intensive care unit for monitoring and treatment. In addition to standard burn evaluation, an electrocardiogram, CBC, and serum chemistry (including creatine phosphokinase and lactic dehydrogenase) should be taken and checked. Myoglobinuria can lead to acute renal failure.

SUGGESTED READING

Reilly DA, Garner WL. Management of chemical injuries to the upper extremity. *Hand Clin.* 2000;16(2):215-224.

Smith MA, Munster AM, Spence RJ. Burns of the hand and upper limb—a review. *Burns.* 1998;24(6):493-505.

Yakuboff KP, Kurtzman LC, Stern PJ. Acute management of thermal and electrical burns of the upper extremity. *Orthop Clin North Am.* 1992;23(1):161-169.

# chapter 36

# FROSTBITE

Frostbite was described by Napoleon's surgeon general in 1812. Although associated with a military history, frostbite is seen in civilians as well. Fingers, toes, face, and ears are most frequently affected. Proper treatment can help salvage tissues and minimize structural and functional loss.

## Mechanism of Injury

- Exposure at 28°F or -2°C causes tissue to freeze.
- Fatigue, dehydration, alcohol or drug use, previous cold injury, wind chill, and water immersion can enhance this process.
- A spectrum of cold injury exists:
  - Frostnip: reversible blanching of tissue
  - Chilblain: recurrent chronic vasculitis from repeated exposures
  - Trench foot (or hand): several hours in cold (10°C to 15°C) and wet area
  - Frostbite: tissue freezes

## Evaluation

- Assess the degree of frostbite:
  - Superficial: skin is supple when palpated, there is minimal tissue loss, the area is painful after rewarming and blisters might form; patients often have resultant permanent cold hypersensitivity.
  - Deep: skin is firm when palpated, there is extensive tissue loss and hyperemic blistering, skin is blue-grey and insensate after rewarming.

- Evaluate the extent of involvement.
- Radiographs should be taken to determine what trauma might have occurred while the limb was anesthetic; children with open growth plates will have growth disturbances.

## Acute Treatment

- Do not rewarm until you are able to keep the patient warm; rewarming and refreezing is more detrimental than delayed treatment.
- The patient's core body temperature should be brought above 35°C.
- Rapidly rewarm affected area in water maintained between 40°C and 42°C for 15 to 30 minutes.
- Administer tetanus prophylaxis.
- Provide appropriate pain management and anti-inflammatories.
- The suggested prophylactic antibiotic regimen is penicillin 600 mg IV every 6 hours for 48 to 72 hours.
- Prohibit use of tobacco (this causes peripheral vasoconstriction).

## Definitive Treatment (Refer to Hand Specialist)

- Clear blisters are debrided, dark are not; aloe vera and sterile dressings are applied.
- The areas are observed for definitive margin of demarcation; prior to surgical intervention, recovery can take as long as 4 weeks.
- Debridement or amputation of necrotic areas is performed.

## Potential Problems

- Infection
- Gangrene
- Pain and cold hypersensitivity
- Growth disturbance
- Osteoporosis/bone loss (focal)

- Skin changes
- Contractures

## Suggested Reading

Su CW, Lohman R, Gottlieb LJ. Frostbite of the upper extremity. *Hand Clin.* 2000;16(2):235-247.

# Appendices

# COMMONLY USED SPLINTS

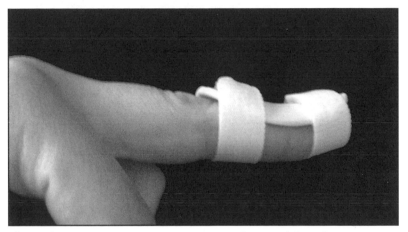

**Figure A-1.** Mallet/DIP joint hyperextension splint immobilizes the DIP joint in hyperextension while leaving the PIP joint free to move.

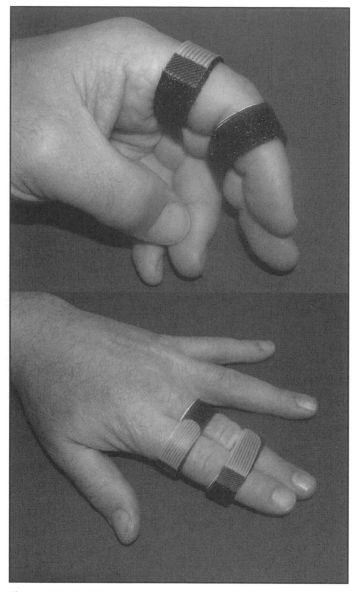

**Figure A-2.** Buddy taping, using either tape or velcro straps, is placed to allow the adjacent finger to serve as a splint, which still allows joint motion.

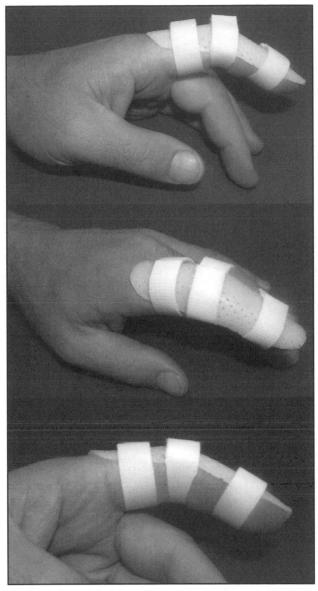

**Figure A-3.** A digital dorsal blocking splint is used to maintain reduction of a PIPJ dislocation or fracture-dislocation; this can be created using an aluminum/foam splint if available.

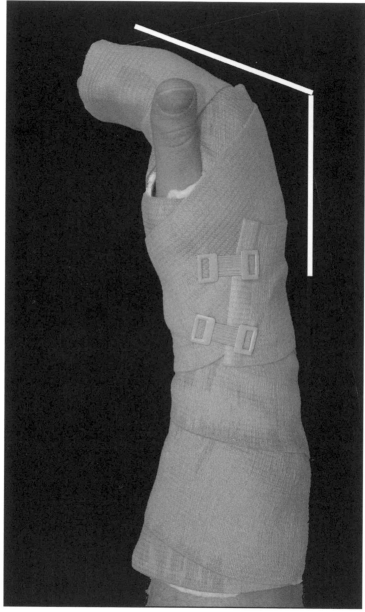

**Figure A-4.** Metacarpal or phalangeal injuries can be immobilized in "neutral," with the MPJs flexed and the IPJs extended.

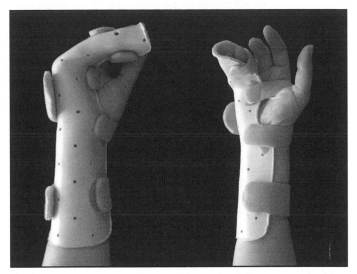

**Figure A-5.** Ulnar gutter splints can be made of plaster or can be fabricated from thermoplast material depending on patient and injury factors.

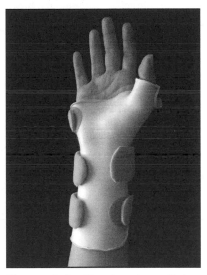

**Figure A-6.** Thumb spica splinting, whether plaster or thermoplast, should immobilize at least the MPJ of the thumb. The IPJ of the thumb sometimes can be left free to move (if the injury does not include the EPL, FPL, IPJ, or distal phalanx).

**Figure A-7.** The standard volar wrist splint should allow full MPJ flexion (fist formation) to prevent stiffness. If supination and pronation must be controlled (both radius and ulna fractures), a sugar tong splint (wrapping around the elbow and extending back to the MPJ dorsally) should be applied.

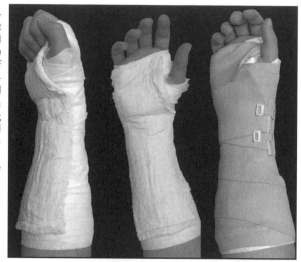

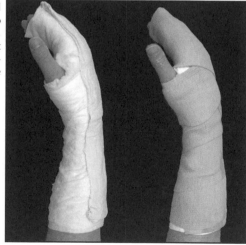

**Figure A-8.** A wrist and digital dorsal block splint can be used to immobilize flexor tendon injuries, preventing extension of the wrist and digit, which can cause retraction of the tendon stump or rupture of repairs.

# DIGITAL ANESTHETIC BLOCK

Four digital nerve branches supply innervations to each digit. There are several reported techniques used to anesthetize these nerves. The authors prefer the dorsal approach, which is less painful for the patient.

You will need:
- Betadine (or equivalent)
- 10 cc syringe filled with 1% lidocaine (no epinephrine)
- 25 gauge needle (~1.5 inches)

1. Prepare the digit and web space with betadine solution.
2. Inject 1 cc wheal of lidocaine in dorsal skin next to extensor tendon and just proximal to web space to anesthetize dorsal digital nerve (Figure B-1A).
3. Insert needle further until it can be seen tenting volar skin. Inject 1 cc lidocaine to block volar digital nerve (Figure B 1B).
4. Withdraw needle to dorsal skin and target it subcutaneously to inject a 1 cc wheal at the dorsal skin on the opposite side of the digit's extensor tendon.
5. Insert needle through wheal on opposite side of extensor tendon as far as the volar digital nerve and inject additional 1 cc lidocaine (Figure B 1C).
6. Wait about 5 minutes for the lidocaine to take effect, then test whether it is working before beginning a procedure.

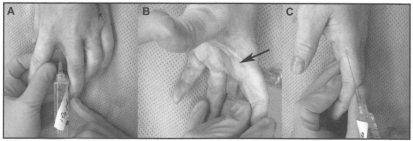

**Figure B-1**

appendix **C**

## TETANUS QUICK REFERENCE

Tetanus is caused by a neurotoxic exotoxin from the anaerobic bacterium *Clostridium tetani*; this affects the central nervous system, causing muscle spasms, seizures, and other potentially fatal sequelae. The bacterium enters the body through contaminated wounds and the incubation period ranges from 3 to 21 days (usually around 8 days). However, tetanus can follow elective surgery, burns, puncture or crush wounds, dental or ear infections, animal bites, abortion, and pregnancy.

CDC Recommendations:* Tetanus immune globulin (TIG) for persons with tetanus helps remove unbound tetanus toxin and is given in a single intramuscular dose of 3000 to 5000 units; part of this is infiltrated around the wound. Intravenous immune globulin (IVIG), which contains tetanus antitoxin, can be used if TIG is not available.

Table C-1*

## TETANUS WOUND MANAGEMENT

| Vaccination History | Clean, Minor Wounds | | Other Wounds | |
|---|---|---|---|---|
| | Td Toxoid | TIG | Td Toxoid | TIG |
| Unknown or <3 Doses | Yes | No | Yes | No |
| 3+ Doses | Only if >10 years since last dose | No | Only if >5 years since last dose | No |

## Table C-2*
# DTAP, DT, TD AND TDAP

|  | Diphtheria | Tetanus |
|---|---|---|
| DTaP, DT | 7 to 8 Lf units | 5 to 12.5 Lf units |
| Td, Tdap (adult) | 2 to 2.5 Lf units | 5 Lf units |

The pediatric Diphtheria-Tetanus-acellular Pertussis (DTaP) vaccine and pediatric Diphtheria-Tetanus (DT) are used through age 6 years.
Adult Tetanus-diphtheria (Td) vaccine is for age 7 and older.
Adult Tetanus-diphtheria-acellular Pertussis (Tdap) is for 10-18 years (Boostrix) or 11-64 years (Adacel).

**Adverse reactions:** Local erythema or induration; systemic reactions are rare.

*From http://www.cdc.gov/vaccines/pubs/pinkbook/downloads/tetanus.pdf

# RABIES QUICK REFERENCE

## Table D-1
## RABIES QUICK REFERENCE

| Vaccination Status | Recommended Treatment Regimen* |
|---|---|
| Not Vaccinated | 1. RIG 20IU/kg body weight (as much as possible around wound, then IM distant from vaccine site)<br>2. Vaccine: HDCV, PCEC, or RVA 1cc IM (deltoid) QD on days 0, 3, 7, 14, 28 |
| Previously Vaccinated and Documented | 1. No RIG<br>2. Vaccine: HDCV or PCEC 1cc IM (deltoid) QD on days 0, 3 only |

*Adapted from http://www.cdc.gov/mmwR/preview/mmwrhtml/rr57e507a1.htm

| | | |
|---|---|---|
| **RIG** | = | Rabies immune globulin |
| **HDCV** | = | Human diploid cell vaccine |
| **RVA** | = | Rabies vaccine adsorbed |
| **PCEC** | = | Purified chick embryo cell vaccine |

# HOW TO REMOVE A TIGHT RING

Rings should be removed at the earliest assessment of a hand injury. If left in place, they can hinder evaluation, obscure radiographic images, and most importantly, lead to loss of the digit if constriction leads to neurovascular compromise.

There are ways to remove tight rings without cutting them. If you have a few minutes and there is no acute neurovascular compromise, a little lubrication with soap and water or surgical lubricant might allow you to twist off the ring. If the ring is too tight, a suture (preferably silk) can be placed under the ring using the needle. The rest of the suture then is used to wrap the digit just distal to the ring to allow it to decrease in size. The suture is used to "slide" the ring further distally on the digit. This can be repeated until the ring is able to be removed (Figure E-1).

In an emergency, a ring cutter should be available (Figure E-2). These can be purchased online for $10-$150. The lip of the ring cutter is inserted between the skin and the ring, and gentle twisting (in the case of a mechanical, rather than electrical ring cutter) will score the ring, eventually cutting it. You can reassure the patient that jewelers usually are able to repair the cut ring.

**Figure E-1.** A suture can be inserted between the skin and the ring and used to wrap the digit in small increments, allowing removal of the ring from the digit.

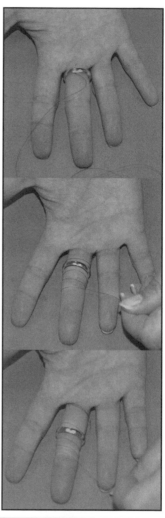

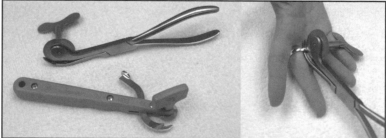

**Figure E-2.** Two examples of ring cutters available. The placement of the lip should be beneath the ring in the area to be cut.

## COMMON HAND INFECTIONS AND BITE WOUNDS

### Table F-1

| Infection | Likely Organism | Initial Antibiotic Agents |
|---|---|---|
| Felon | *Staphylococcus aureus* or streptococci | First-generation cephalosporin or penicillin (anti-staphylococcal) |
| Paronychia | *Staphylococcus aureus*, or streptococci (polymicrobial or gram negative if oral exposure, *C. albicans* if chronic) | First-generation cephalosporin or penicillin (anti-staphylococcal); if gram negative suspected, can use clindamycin |
| Infectious Tenosynovitis | *Staphylococcus aureus*, streptococci, anaerobes; consider *Neisseria gonorrhoeae* | Beta-lactamase inhibitor (ampicillin-sulbactam) IV<br>If possible *N. gonorrhoeae* ceftriaxone or fluoroquinolone IV |
| Bites:<br> Cat or dog<br><br><br> Human | *Pasteurella multocida*, *S. aureus*, *Pseudomona*, and *Streptococcus*<br><br>*S. aureus*, streptococci, *Eikenella corrodens*, gram-negative bacilli, anaerobes | Beta-lactamase inhibitor (ampicillin-sulbactam) or second-generation cephalosporin (cefoxitin), PO amoxicillin/clavulanate on discharge |
| Herpetic Whitlow | HSV 1 and HSV 2 | Consider antivirals if <48 hours or recurrent, antimicrobials only if secondarily infected |

## TREATMENT OF COMMON CHEMICAL BURNS

### Table G-1

| Agent | Usual Source | Important Labs | Management |
|-------|-------------|----------------|------------|
| Acidic Agents | | | |
| Chromic Acid | Used for electroplating. Enters bloodstream and binds to hemoglobin, impairing oxygenation. Causes GI hemorrhage, liver failure, and coagulopathies. | Renal, liver function, blood count | Water irrigation, phosphate buffer, or 5% thiosulfate soaks; topical 10% calcium EDTA ointment; dimercaprol, ascorbic acid, or sodium calcium edentate |
| Formic Acid | Industrial agent. Can cause systemic acidosis (both metabolic and respiratory) and organ failure. | Vitals (BP), CBC, chemistry, UA, ABG (acidosis) | Water irrigation, IV hydration/bicarbonate, folic acid |

*Continued*

## Table G-1
### Continued

| Agent | Usual Source | Important Labs | Management |
|-------|-------------|----------------|------------|
| Acidic Agents: | | | |
| Hydrofluoric Acid | Usually found in industrial solvents, cleaners, fertilizers. The anhydrous form is strong and causes severe immediate tissue destruction. The aqueous form is weak and causes burn over several hours. Deep and superficial burns can develop. Also can cause severe systemic metabolic problems. | Vitals, cardiac monitor, chemistry | Water 20 minutes; benzalkonium choloride irrigation, calcium gluconate gels until pain resolution; 10% calcium gluconate injection (0.5cc/cm$^2$) at periphery of burn |
| Monochloroacetic Acid | Used as an herbicide, also as a wart remover in Europe. Affects cellular energy cycle, causing lactic acidosis. Can cause systemic lethal poisoning. | Cardiac monitor, chemistry, lactate | Dichloroacetate (DCA) if greater than 5% BSA (reduces lactic acid accumulation) |

Continued

## Table G-1
### Continued

| Agent | Usual Source | Important Labs | Management |
|---|---|---|---|
| Acidic Agents: | | | |
| Phenol (Weak Acid) | Primarily used in medicine (chemical peels, nerve injections). Causes denaturing of proteins. Anesthetic properties, so patient might not feel damage occurring. Can cause cardiac arrhythmias, CNS depression, and organ issues. | CBC, glucose, electrolytes, peripheral blood smear, urinalysis, and/or hemoglobin/haptoglobin to assess hemolysis | Decontaminate with 50% polyethylene glycol (PEG) and water irrigation |
| Alkali Agents: | | | |
| Airbag Injury | Sodium azide and sodium hydroxide burns accompany thermal injury as well as abrasion from release of talcum. | | Water irrigation, treat thermal injury |
| Ammonia | Anhydrous form is in drain and oven cleaners. Causes liquifactive necrosis with a freeze injury as well, due to storage at low temperatures. Can be accompanied by inhalation or ocular injury. | | Water irrigation (or soap and water), then treat as thermal burn |

Continued

## Table G-1
*Continued*

| Agent | Usual Source | Important Labs | Management |
|-------|-------------|----------------|------------|
| Alkali Agents: | | | |
| Black Liquor | Used to make pulp (for paper) out of wood chips; it is a heated mixture of sodium bicarbonate, sodium sulfide, sodium thiosulfate, and sodium sulfate. | | Water irrigation, treat thermal injury |
| Cement Burns | Mixture of calcium oxide and silicon oxide. Causes liquefactive necrosis (contact), thermal burns (from heat), and/or explosive burns. Commonly progress to full thickness burns over 12 to 48 hours of exposure. | | Remove with cloth, soap, and copious running water |
| Povidine-iodine (Betadine) | Can cause burns in body creases or under tourniquet. | | Water irrigation, remove Betadine |

*Continued*

## Table G-1
### Continued

| Agent | Usual Source | Important Labs | Management |
|---|---|---|---|
| Sulfur Mustard | Vesicant (blistering agent) used in chemical warfare. Causes inflammation, DNA cross-linking, cholinergic activity. Blistering from 48 hours to 2 weeks after exposure. Can compromise airway, cause GI distress, and suppress hematopoiesis. | CBC for several weeks; monitor for several hours as symptoms might not occur for hours to days following exposure | Decontamination with water must occur within 1 to 2 minutes; once patient arrives to emergency center, the damage has already been done and decontamination is aimed at protecting medical personnel. There is no antidote. Medical management is supportive. |
| White Phosphorus | Oxidizing agent used in fireworks, weaponry, fertilizers. Autoignites at 30°C, oxidizes on skin until neutralized, debrided, or consumed. Causes painful yellowish burn. Can cause metabolic issues (calcium/phosphate levels). | Chemistry (Ca, Phos), hepatic and renal function, cardiac monitor | Thorough water irrigation, cover wound with wet compresses (prevent ignition), surgical removal of agent |

*Also refer to the Agency for Toxic Substances and Disease Registry (of the Center for Disease Control). Visit the website at: http://www.atsdr.cdc.gov/

## *ORTHOPEDIC ABBREVIATIONS*

### Digits

| | |
|---|---|
| **Th** | Thumb |
| **IF** | Index finger |
| **LF** | Long finger |
| **RF** | Ring finger |
| **SF** | Small finger |

### Anatomic Structures

| | |
|---|---|
| **AdP** | Adductor pollicis |
| **APB** | Abductor pollicis brevis |
| **CMC** | Carpal metacarpal |
| **CMCJ** | Carpal metacarpal joint |
| **DIO** | Dorsal interosseous (muscle) |
| **DIP** | Distal interphalangeal |
| **DIPJ** | Distal interphalangeal joint |
| **ECRB** | Extensor carpi radialis brevis |
| **ECRL** | Extensor carpi radialis longus |
| **ECU** | Extensor carpi ulnaris |
| **EDC** | Extensor digitorum communis |
| **EDQ** | Extensor digiti quinti |
| **EDM** | Extensor digiti minimi |
| **EIP** | Extensor indices proprius |
| **EPB** | Extensor pollicis brevis |
| **EPL** | Extensor pollicis longus |
| **FCR** | Flexor carpi radialis |
| **FCU** | Flexor carpi ulnaris |
| **FDP** | Flexor digitorum profundus |

| | |
|---|---|
| **FDS** | Flexor digitorum superficialis |
| **FPL** | Flexor pollicis longus |
| **IP** | Interphalangeal |
| **IPJ** | Interphalangeal joint |
| **MCP** | Metacarpophalangeal |
| **MCPJ** | Metacarpophalangeal joint |
| **OP** | Opponens pollicis |
| **PIP** | Proximal interphalangeal |
| **PIPJ** | Proximal interphalangeal joint |
| **PL** | Palmaris longus |

## Procedures

| | |
|---|---|
| **CR** | Closed reduction |
| **CRPP** | Closed reduction, percutaneous pinning |
| **EF** | External fixation |
| **I&D** | Irrigation and debridement (or incision and drainage) |
| **IF** | Internal fixation |
| **OR** | Open reduction |
| **ORIF** | Open reduction, internal fixation |
| **PP** | Percutaneous pinning |

# HAND EXAMINATION DIAGRAM TEMPLATE

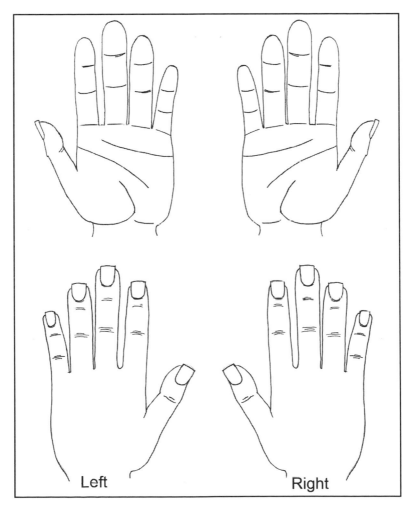

Left                    Right

# MOTOR/SENSORY NERVE QUICK REFERENCE

## Table J-1

| Nerve | Muscle Innervation | Sensory Innervation |
|-------|--------------------|--------------------|
| Median | Flexor carpi radialis<br>Palmaris longus<br>Flexor digitorum superficialis<br>Flexor digitorum profundus (index and long)<br>Flexor pollicis longus<br>Lumbricals 1,2<br>Opponens pollicis<br>Flexor pollicis brevis (radial 1/2)<br>Abductor pollicis brevis | Radial aspect of palm (palmar cutaneous branch)<br>Thumb, index, long, and radial half of ring fingers |
| Ulnar | Flexor carpi ulnaris<br>Flexor digitorum profundus (ring and small)<br>Lumbricals 3,4<br>Interossei<br>Adductor pollicis<br>Flexor pollicis brevis (ulnar 1/2)<br>Abductor digiti minimi | Small finger and ulnar half of ring finger |

*Continued*

## Table J-1
*Continued*

| Nerve | Muscle Innervation | Sensory Innervation |
|-------|--------------------|--------------------|
| Radial | Extensor carpi radialis brevis<br>Extensor carpi radialis longus<br>Extensor carpi ulnaris<br>Extensor digitorum communis<br>Extensor indices proprius<br>Extensor pollicis longus<br>Extensor pollicis brevis<br>Abductor pollicis longus | Dorsum of hand (superficial branch) |

# INDEX

# WAIT
## ...*There's More!*

### Curbside Consultation of the Shoulder: 49 Clinical Questions
Gregory Nicholson, MD; Matthew Provencher, MD
176 pp., Soft Cover, 2008,
ISBN 13: 978-1-55642-827-2, Order #18278, **$79.95**

*Curbside Consultation of the Shoulder: 49 Clinical Questions* provides information basic enough for residents while also incorporating expert advice that even high-volume clinicians will appreciate. Practicing orthopedic surgeons, orthopedic residents, and medical students will benefit from the user-friendly and casual format and the expert advice contained within.

### Biologic Joint Reconstruction: Alternatives to Joint Arthroplasty
Brian Cole, MD; Andreas Gomoll, MD
250 pp., Soft Cover, 2009
ISBN 13: 978-1-55642-850-0, Order #18500, **$149.95**

*Biologic Joint Reconstruction* is the only orthopedic text on the market that combines discussion of biological and limited prosthetic options for the treatment of chondral damage and early arthritis for the young active adult, as well as for traditional joint replacement patients.

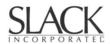